D0255655

Guilt-free Bottle-feeding

993467502_1

WITHDRAWN

Guilt-free Bottle-feeding

Why your formula-fed baby *can* be happy, healthy and smart

Madeleine Morris
With Dr Sasha Howard

white
LADDER

Important note

The information in this book is not intended as a substitute for medical advice. Neither the author nor White Ladder can accept any responsibility for any injury, damages or losses suffered as a result of following the information herein.

Guilt-free Bottle-feeding: Why your formula-fed baby can be happy, healthy and smart

This first edition published in 2014 by White Ladder Press, an imprint of Crimson Publishing Ltd, 19–21c Charles Street, Bath BA1 1HX.

© Madeleine Morris 2014
Cover photo of Madeleine Morris © Lucy J Toms Photography

The right of Madeleine Morris to be identified as the author of this work has been asserted by her in accordance with the Copyright, Designs and Patents Act 1988.

All rights reserved. This book is sold subject to the condition that it shall not, by way of trade or otherwise, be lent, resold, hired out or otherwise circulated without the publisher's prior written consent in any form of binding or cover other than that in which it is published and without a similar condition including this condition being imposed on the subsequent purchaser. No part of this publication may be reproduced, stored in a retrieval system or transmitted in any form or by any means, electronic and mechanical, photocopying, recording or otherwise without prior permission of Crimson Publishing Ltd.

British Library Cataloguing in Publication Data
A catalogue record for this book is available from the British Library.

ISBN 978 1 908281 77 7

Typeset by IDSUK (DataConnections) Ltd
Printed and bound in Malta by Gutenberg Press Ltd, Malta

For my mother, who gave me everything, and for my daughter, who gave me everything else.

Madeleine Morris

To my daughter, my husband, and my mum.

Dr Sasha Howard

GLOUCESTERSHIRE COUNTY COUNCIL	
9934675021	
Bertrams	30/10/2014
AN	£10.99
GMO	

Contents

Foreword ix

About the authors xi

Acknowledgements xiii

Introduction 1

Part 1: The theory

1 Why mothers bottle-feed 17

2 Why bottle-feeding will not make your baby fat,
 sick or stupid 44

3 The Breastfeeding Echo Chamber: how everything
 you read reinforces 'breast is best' 77

4 Guilt, pressure and support 115

Conclusion: The view in our toddler-shaped rear-view
mirrors 148

Part 2: The practice

1 Choosing a formula 155

2 Choosing a bottle 173

3 Sterilising 177

4 Preparing a feed 180

Contents

5 Feeding   185

6 Switching from breast to bottle   194

7 Common bottle-feeding side effects and problems   197

Resources   201

Endnotes   205

Foreword

For many, the journey into parenthood is a time filled with hopes and expectations. Surrounded by soft images and emotive messages, new and expectant parents begin to build their hopes, dreams and ideals of what becoming a mother or father will be like. They build their aspirations of bringing a new child or children into the world to love, teach and grow into unique people of their own.

But, sometimes unbeknownst to them, these hopes and aspirations are constantly being developed and reinforced by 'perfect' mother and baby images that pervade media portrayals of motherhood, together with stories of celebrity motherhood bliss. Images typically reflect a perfect mother, in control, who is able to conceive and give birth naturally and breastfeed her baby.

This places enormous pressure on women to try to live up to these images, despite the reality that often becoming parents, and parenthood itself, is filled with many, ongoing, challenges. There are specific milestones along the way to becoming a parent, such as conception and birth, that pose additional challenges for some, though not for others. These challenges and disappointments are generally not spoken about openly, depriving parents of support at a time when they need it most.

This whole notion of ideals, expectations and pressures applies even more to the issue of breastfeeding. There is still a lot of spoken and unspoken pressure and criticism surrounding how we feed our children, and whether we are 'good' and 'natural' mothers who are truly 'giving their child the best start' by breastfeeding.

Given that women are more likely to develop depression and anxiety in the period before and after the birth of a child than at any other time of their lives, the impact of these pressures on maternal mental health is significant. Pressure, judgements and often unspoken criticism commonly lead women, who may already be extremely disappointed in themselves, to feel worse, as though they have failed as individuals, and as mothers.

Like the cases described in this book, my own research with women who have experienced postnatal depression reveals that mothers spontaneously describe either real or perceived pressure from family and health professionals to continue to breastfeed when they are struggling, and they describe great sadness and grief at not being able to do so for a variety of reasons. Most critically, the woman with postnatal depression or anxiety is convinced she is the *only* one to fall short of this ideal, and she feels she is a failure compared with other mothers, and compared with her expectations of herself.

While it is important to reinforce the health benefits of breastfeeding, we need to stop and consider the impact of health promotion messages and professional advice, policies and practices on those who may not be in a position to breastfeed successfully.

This book is an excellent step towards doing just that – bridging the gap between the ideals and realities of breastfeeding and bottle-feeding. It provides women, for the first time, with high-quality evidence that does not negate the benefits of breastfeeding, but, importantly, portrays the realistic backdrop to many of our aspirations and ideals.

To date, these facts have not been spelled out clearly for women, which has led to endless unnecessary pressure, grief, guilt and disappointment surrounding bottle-feeding.

Guilt-free Bottle-feeding is not only easy to read and well written, but, importantly, it is full of facts that will give parents the real story, the full story. By doing this, I believe this book will make a great contribution to reducing the unnecessary shame, guilt and failure that currently exist surrounding bottle-feeding, and, more broadly, will help us build the much-needed momentum towards the creation of a more realistic, sensitive and honest culture surrounding motherhood for our parents of tomorrow.

Dr Nicole Highet
Founder and Executive Director
COPE: Centre of Perinatal Excellence

About the authors

Madeleine Morris is an award-winning journalist and broadcaster. During her 12-year career with the BBC, Madeleine reported from more than 20 countries, including the USA, where she was a correspondent in 2010. In 2012 she won the One World Media Award for best radio documentary for an investigation into the micro-finance industry in India. Madeleine has spent a considerable part of her career reporting from and on the developing world, and she was a founding trustee of the African children's charity Dramatic Need. She has written for *The Times*, *Guardian*, *Sydney Morning Herald* and the *Age*.

Madeleine and her husband moved back to their native Australia in 2012 to be closer to family and to raise their daughter in the sunshine. She currently reports for the ABC (Australian Broadcasting Corporation). This is her first book.

Sasha Howard is a paediatrician with a special interest in paediatric endocrinology. Sasha has worked in the NHS for 10 years and is currently also writing a PhD thesis in the field of childhood growth and development. She has professional experience of looking after many newborn infants and new mothers learning to feed their babies, and is also a mum to a young daughter.

In her work she has seen first-hand the difficulties many mothers and babies face when breastfeeding. She herself struggled to breastfeed her daughter, and experienced the pain and guilt many mothers face when considering the choice to bottle-feed their baby.

Sasha is the author of several peer-reviewed scientific papers and book chapters and has presented her academic work internationally.

www.guiltfreebottlefeeding.com

Acknowledgements

This book owes a huge intellectual debt to several people. Firstly, to Joan Wolf, who did such groundbreaking, brave work examining the evidence behind breastfeeding recommendations. Her ideas on total motherhood greatly influenced not only this book but my life, and I am very grateful. Secondly, Suzanne Barston, aka the Fearless Formula Feeder, has been another intellectual leader and emotional support in discussions around bottle-feeding. As well as being smart and brave, her generosity of spirit as I have gone through the process of writing has been incredible. All of us formula-feeders are lucky to have such a warm, caring soul as a team leader. Ellie Lee and her team at the University of Kent have led the way on more nuanced discussions of feeding and parenting in general. Lisa Watson and the incredible team at Bottle Babies have provided invaluable support in sourcing contributors, and Lisa gave much-needed feedback and advice on the drafts. You guys do such a wonderful job supporting women for no reward other than satisfaction. Thank you.

Huge thanks to my agent, Jane Graham Maw, for her dogged belief in this project; to Hugh Brune, my publisher at Crimson for picking it up; and to Beth Bishop, my editor, for all her work to make it a better book. Muchas gracias to my other test readers – Sam, Margot Morris, Sophie, Sue Battersby – for suggestions and improvements. Thank you to my other contributors: Katie Hinde, Janet Fyle, Mandy Belfort, David Lancy, Lenore Skenazy, Brooke Scelza, Polly Palumbo, Hilary Mercer, Kate Kripke, Karleen Gribble and Charlotte Faircloth. Thanks to Helen Crawley and the First Steps Nutrition Trust for their wonderful work on providing thorough, unbiased information on formula. Thank you to Dr Nicole Highet for writing the foreword and for your incredible commitment to helping mums. Many thanks to the women, and one man, who have shared their stories here in the hope they will help others. Recalling those hard times has been painful for many of you. I am so very grateful that you braved that pain for us.

My great thanks to my dear friend and co-author Dr Sasha Howard, without whose input this book would not exist. Thank you for being brave enough to come on this journey with me, and for all your late nights, wisdom and experience. Thanks also to Fang Fang, Erlinda, Lisa and Lisa, the wonderful women who got us through those first life-changing months as new mums. We love you guys.

To all my friends and family, near and far, who have supported this project from its inception – there are too many of you to name, but I am so grateful for your encouragement and belief.

Deepest thanks to my parents-in-law, Archie and Mary Lou, who have supported us in so many ways. My thanks to my wonderful parents. My mother, who flew from Australia to look after our baby for a month so I could go to the British Library and see if there was something to this idea for a book, and has continued her unwavering support, both emotionally and practically. My father, who has never had anything but the most unshakeable belief in me, in any endeavour. There are no words for everything you have both given to all three of your daughters. I hope this book goes some way to honouring that sacrifice and belief.

Thanks to my beautiful daughter, who has given me more than I could ever have understood or imagined.

And finally to my husband, Sam. Thank you for your unwavering support. For all the hours you've looked after our baby on your own so I could work. For giving me the space, and the financial liberty, to pursue something I was passionate about. For the laughs, more than a decade in. You are the very definition of a true life partner. I love you, I am so grateful to you, and I promise to do my share of the washing-up from now on.

Madeleine Morris, 30 January 2014

Introduction

It's 2 a.m., 27 September 2011. The postnatal ward is washed in the bluey-green glow of exit signs and blinking machines. I'm lying in my second-best pyjamas, my pants stuffed with the world's biggest maternity pad, eyes heavy with bags that tell of a nine-hour labour, a litre of blood loss and nearly 40 hours continuously awake. Beside me, in a plastic crib, is the scrawny, 7lb ½oz light of my life, my new daughter. And she won't shut up.

As her mewling turns to squeaking rage, my efforts at feeding, rocking, patting and comforting seem more and more futile. Despite my lack of experience and sleep, I understand what is wrong. She is hungry. She is hungry, even though she spent what seemed like most of her first 20 hours at my breast. She is hungry, even though my nipples are already red-raw, and my boobs are so enormous they could star in their own porn film. She is hungry, even though the well-meaning maternity nurse tells me she's probably just suckling for comfort.

Desperate to placate her, a nagging thought worms its way into my mushy brain. 'What if I just give her a little bit of formula? Just to fill her tummy so she can get to sleep?' (I had had a breast reduction many years before so was prepared not to be able to breastfeed at all. When I started leaking colostrum in the shower a few weeks before my daughter arrived I was pleasantly surprised.)

I quickly bat the thought away. 'Breast is best' after all, and I know that breastfeeding might take some time to establish. But as the minutes tick by, and she becomes hoarse from heartbreaking squeaks, I make a decision. Gingerly, I get out of bed, hobble down the corridor to the nurses' station and ask for a bottle of formula. The young midwife looks a little harried, asks if I'm sure, and when I respond that I am, she says she can get a bottle for me. I just have to sign The Form.

Ahhh... The Form. The Form tells me that my hospital follows the UNICEF Baby Friendly Initiative, which supports and protects breastfeeding, step 6 of which is: 'Give newborn infants no food or drink other than breast milk, unless clinically indicated.' It then proceeds to give me a list of what might happen if I choose to ignore The Sixth Commandment.

I may experience, among other things, 'delay in milk coming in, reduced milk supply, baby less likely to be breastfed, more likely to stop breastfeeding earlier than intended, the use of a teat may confuse your baby, introducing larger volumes of milk which stretch the stomach, baby may then appear less satisfied when breastfed, protection against infection and allergies is reduced'.

It is essentially saying: 'Lady, if you slip up once and give that baby a bottle, kiss goodbye to any chance of successful breastfeeding. If it doesn't work out, it will be your fault.' And if you don't breastfeed, we all know what that means – you're a bad mum. The Form is clearly designed to inspire fear, and it's doing its job perfectly.

My daughter is exhausted. I'm exhausted. She's ravenously hungry. What do I do?

It's a dilemma faced by thousands of women all over the world every day, and not only at the very beginning of their child's life. Inundated by a barrage of anti-formula 'education', but unsuccessful at breastfeeding and desperate for an alternative, do we follow the official advice and keep the boobs in business, no matter what the cost to our own well-being, or the cost to our baby? Or do we succumb to the lure of the bottle, and all the judgement and guilt that come with it?

Rewind 60 years and breastfeeding seemed to be on its way out. A medicalised view of childbirth told mothers that the best they could do for their baby, to 'make sure he was getting enough', was to start him immediately on a bottle. Newborns were also kept in separate, centralised nurseries so mothers could recover and women were often sedated during childbirth. (Actually, that last one has some appeal. Admit it. I'd never do it, obviously, but there were certainly moments of my labour when I longed for someone to knock me out.)

By the early 1950s, only around a quarter of American women were giving breastfeeding a go immediately after birth,[1] and about half of new British mothers.[2] Appalled at this state of affairs, and driven by their religious belief that God had intended women to breastfeed, a group of Catholic Chicagoans got together in 1958 to form La Leche League and set about reviving what seemed to be a dying art.

Leap forward 60 years and what started in the front room of a devout housewife has become a co-ordinated, global campaign, with international frameworks and policies, thousands of support groups, scores of annual conferences and millions of government dollars all aimed at encouraging women to do what their breasts were designed to do – feed their young.

And thank goodness. Had we lost the practice and art of breastfeeding, it would have been a monumental travesty, a denial of a basic human function that makes millions of women and babies happy and keeps those babies nourished every day.

And yet, and yet … While this much-needed campaign brought breastfeeding back from the brink, the majority of women in the West will still, at some stage, feed their babies formula. And because the pro-breastfeeding message has become synonymous with a virulent anti-formula dogma, that makes us feel guilty.

That's exactly how I felt just minutes after I signed The Form in hospital that night, put a bottle in my newborn daughter's mouth, and watched her greedily gulp down 10 millilitres before immediately dropping into a blissful sleep.

As she dozed, shame washed over me. How could I have already condemned my perfect little baby to a second-class life, less than 24 hours into my journey into motherhood, just because I wasn't strong enough to make it through the tough times? She would get sick. She would get fat. She would be stupid, all because I was weak and selfish and a bad mother. I should have just gritted my teeth and let her keep sucking no matter how much it hurt or how tired I was, or how hungry she seemed to be. I had been 'booby-trapped' already.

Sadly, this is where decades of the 'breast is best', anti-formula message has got us: not a tribe of mothers happily nursing our young, but a splintered gaggle who define our success at motherhood by how we feed our babies.

After a steady climb since the low points of the 1970s, breastfeeding rates are now increasing only slowly. In the UK, around 80% of British mothers initially try, but by the time a baby is one week old,

If you are reading this book before deciding whether to breastfeed or not, we would encourage you to give it a go. You may like it more than you thought you would. You might also be one of those lucky ones who find it to be the easiest and most convenient thing in the world, and, all other things being equal, breast milk is nutritionally the better option.

If you're struggling with breastfeeding and want to continue, we strongly encourage you to get proper help and advice. In many cases it really can make all the difference. There's a list of places you can go for help in the resources section.

And if you have decided you don't want to breastfeed from the outset, or you have already tried your damnedest and know you're ready to stop, or you've been using formula but feeling guilty for doing so, then welcome. This book is for you. It's not written for academics; it doesn't seek to quote every feminist work on the politics of the female body and reproduction. It's not written for policy makers, midwives or doctors; it's not a systematic review of every piece of breastfeeding literature published in the last decade. *Guilt-free Bottle-feeding* is written for ordinary, intelligent mums and dads who have found themselves caught between a much-vaunted ideal and the reality of feeding a baby in the modern, developed world.

Please don't use this book to fuel the breast versus bottle debate. The argument is simplistic and stupid, and the only victims are mothers who, quite frankly, have enough on their plate already. It is a great shame that in the quest to encourage more women to breastfeed, bottle-feeding has become demonised. Let's not make the same mistake when removing the stigma from formula. Every parent should actively support a woman's right to breastfeed wherever and whenever she wants, without judgement. The same applies to bottle-feeding.

Why we've written *Guilt-free Bottle-feeding*

You might be wondering what qualifies us, a journalist and a paediatrician, to write this book. After all, we aren't midwives, we haven't helped hundreds of women learn to bottle-feed and we aren't researchers in infant feeding.

Sasha and I met in our NCT antenatal class in London. It quickly became very apparent to me that she knew a lot more about this baby business than our drippy teacher, who told us how *she* thought we should give birth, based on her own personal ideology, rather than giving us the facts and letting us make our own decisions.

Sasha and I quickly became firm friends, and after our daughters were born, we, and the rest of our fantastic mothers' group, met every Tuesday for (decaf) coffee and a sanity-saving debrief. Unsurprisingly, feeding was the main topic of conversation, along with the usual poop and sleep. Not one single one of us had an easy breastfeeding experience, and, like the majority of British mums, by the end of the first month many of us were guiltily topping up with formula.

As a journalist, I value facts above all else. As a paediatrician and research scientist, Sasha does too.

And so it was that I began to wonder how a group of such smart, loving mothers of such longed-for, beautiful babies could all be doing something so harmful. And I wondered how so many children I knew, me included, who were predominantly reared on formula could turn out to be healthy, smart and happy, if formula was poison. So I started to research breastfeeding and bottle-feeding. And, helped by the seminal work of some brave researchers and writers, I discovered that the benefits of breastfeeding are far more nuanced, and likely far smaller, than what our antenatal teacher had told me, and I began to see how so much of the guilt that bottle-feeding mums feel is ill-founded.

And that made me angry. I was angry because I saw so many of my friends tying themselves into pretzels to breastfeed, with no thought for their own well-being, because they felt so pressured. I saw my other friends who'd already stopped breastfeeding wrestling with formula guilt and questions over bottle-feeding because there was no one to offer help or advice. And I got really angry when I saw my friend develop postnatal depression, at least partially caused by the intensive breastfeeding routine she was put on at her 'Baby Friendly' hospital, which saw her not sleep for five days after a horrendous birth. That last one made me *really* angry.

So I decided to do something about it, and I asked Sasha to join me.

All the information presented to you in this book to back up our case that you can rear a happy, healthy, intelligent baby on formula is already in the scientific literature. Sasha has used her skills as a children's doctor and a researcher to check and double-check what the science is really saying. My job, learned through 15 years on the front line as an award-winning journalist, is to put it all together in a way that cuts through the ideologically driven b.s. that counts for so much parenting advice these days.

What we offer you are two fastidious researchers who have come to the same conclusion that so many working with children will voice privately – that breastfeeding is great if it works, but that formula is a pretty damned good alternative. The difference is, we're prepared to say it.

How my own story panned out

So, what about my own guilt? Well, the morning after that first night in hospital, I woke up with a new resolve: I was going to get back on the exclusive breastfeeding horse. Good mothers breastfeed, after all, and having fallen head over heels for my beautiful baby girl, I was determined to be the best mother ever.

I was assisted in my mission by an extremely perky breastfeeding counsellor (her outlook, I mean, not her breasts) who came around with her hand-knitted boob and eagerly demonstrated The Latch. With my husband, my mother and my sister looking on, my daughter and I practised latching as though our lives depended on it. Hers did, I suppose. After approving nods from the counsellor and the nurses, our little family went home.

Over the next week our delirious happiness alternated with delirium as feeding our baby took centre stage in our lives. I'd sit on the couch, glass of water at my side, pillows strategically placed, and put her to my massive mammaries 10 to 14 times a day. As my toes curled up with the initial pain, she would suck, and suck and suck, sometimes for an hour or more. But even though she was at my breast for a good part of the day, she was still losing weight.

The community midwives would come over every two days, as is the norm in Britain, which is where I gave birth, watch as she fed, tell me my latch looked good and tick a mental, if not actual, box. When I mentioned my previous breast surgery and wondered aloud if she was getting enough food, no one seemed that concerned. I was told to keep going, that my 'milk would come in soon', and above all not to fall back into the trap I had strayed into in hospital and give her some formula.

As that first week progressed, my husband and I developed a fear of the dark. Every night as the sun fell we would pray that this would be the night she wouldn't cry inconsolably between midnight and 5 a.m., as we took turns trying to comfort her, with me periodically putting her to the breast. Every morning we would wake up, eyes heavier than the day before, and wonder what we were doing wrong. Was it colic? Something more serious? My mother told us she was probably 'just getting used to the world' and would soon settle down, but I had my doubts.

Then, on day six, the midwife weighed my daughter, saw she had lost 13% of her birth weight, watched her perfectly good latch, listened to my story about the surgery and said, 'I think you should top her up with formula.' It was all we needed – the medical okay to do what we had instinctively wanted to do, but had been too scared to. Lo and behold, that night she fed and slept and fed and slept, breast topped up by bottle each time, without raging tears. What she had been trying to tell us all along, through all those dark hours, was that she was hungry.

My guilt at having given her the devil formula was overtaken a thousand-fold by guilt at not having listened to my instinct, to my clearly hungry baby, and just damn well given her a bottle. To this day, I still wince when I think about my perfect, hungry little girl, and me listening to a flawed ideology instead of her.

We soon got into a routine familiar to many: breast for 40 minutes to an hour followed by bottle top-up eight to 10 times a day, plus expressing morning, noon and night. Ah, the glamour of sitting suctioned to a very expensive milking machine, counting the pitiful droplets as they leached out of my useless breasts. This was why I became a mother!

Nearly two months after my daughter was born, I looked up from the dent I had made in the couch and reassessed. I was rapidly tiring of watching life go by, while I did very little else other than repeat the endless, drudging cycle in pursuit of a never-increasing supply of milk. Breastfeeding was not bonding me to my baby, it was bonding me to my pyjamas. Bolstered by my research into breastfeeding and bottle-feeding, I made another decision. I decided to spend these precious moments of my daughter's early life simply enjoying and getting to know her, instead of obsessing over how much I'd pumped that day, and whether 40 minutes on each breast was enough. I chose our relationship, and my sanity, over breastfeeding. I shed a tear as I told her it didn't mean I loved her any less, poured myself a large glass of Chardonnay, packed away the boobs and the expressing machine, and didn't look back.

My daughter is now a healthy, delightfully happy toddler, who couldn't be more bonded to both me and my husband. She's tall like me, is of average weight and I think she's pretty smart, for a kid who thinks Cookie Monster lives behind her ear.

Authors' notes

- *Guilt-free Bottle-feeding* presumes that formula is what you're putting in the bottle, as it's the milk itself that is typically the source of the guilt, not the bottle. If you are exclusively expressing and bottle-feeding expressed milk, there could be a number of other challenges which we won't go into here. By all means, keep reading, but if you're looking for help specifically with issues relating to expressing, storing breast milk and any associated emotions and practicalities, please take a look at the resources section for organisations that will be able to help you better.
- Just to be absolutely clear: we have never been, and will never be, sponsored by, paid by, affiliated to or in any way in bed with formula companies or any company that manufactures anything to do with bottle-feeding. They've given us nothing – no free samples, no money, not even a cup of tea. In researching this book we have not communicated with any formula companies or formula industry groups. Any information credited to them comes from material already freely available on the internet.
- Also, please note that the medical studies, personal stories and media examples used here all come from the developed world. There are good reasons why breastfeeding is the preferred method in countries where clean water and sanitation aren't freely available,

formula is relatively much more costly and breast milk's protective qualities against some infections are much more important. We have also only looked at studies into healthy, full-term infants, as babies born prematurely or with serious illness have special needs that can't be discussed within the scope of this book. If this describes your baby and you are having trouble breastfeeding or don't want to, please discuss it with your health professional.

- Throughout this book we use the pronoun 'she' when referring to babies. This is because we like girls more. Just kidding – it's because we both have girls, and we have to choose to refer to one gender for the sake of clarity. The content obviously refers to boys as well.

by a screaming baby and your fear that you were starving her. Your bank balance may have made the choice for you – you needed to go back to work and you couldn't or didn't want to manage the pumping. For some of you, pouring that first bottle of formula may have felt like a relief – you didn't really want to breastfeed in the first place but you felt you should. But just because you were relieved doesn't mean you can't also feel guilty.

There are so many reasons that we end up bottle-feeding – physical, institutional and psychological – and we're going to look at some of them here. But before we do that, let's just be crystal clear on two points. Firstly, you do *not* need to have a reason not to breastfeed. We are not at school. There is nothing compulsory about this. You don't have to get a note from your parents. It's your body, your baby. (And for anyone who whines at you, 'but your poor baby has no choice', I suggest you remind them that that's what parenting is – making choices for babies because they can't do so themselves, *because they are babies*. Their baby had no choice about having a judgemental arsehat for a parent, either.) Secondly, the circumstances that lead parents to choose bottles are individual to every family. There is no checklist, so please do not think that if your own path to bottle-feeding isn't written here it is somehow less 'valid'.

How many *really* can't breastfeed? (It depends who you ask)

If you've ever looked up anything breast-related on the internet, you'll have seen the oft-touted statistic: 'Only 1% to 5% of women physically can't breastfeed.' And if you're like me, your jaw will have dropped the first time you read it. Really? I mean, REALLY??? How is it that every single one of my mothers' group friends had breastfeeding problems? Are we all just unluckily in that 5%? Or have we just been 'booby-trapped' into *thinking* we can't? Oh, that's right. We're just *not trying hard enough*. Of course. It's our fault, and what's more we're lying about it. Bad mummies!

Touting this statistic willy-nilly is damaging to mothers. It's sheer finger-pointing and blame dressed up as incontrovertible scientific fact, which serves no purpose other than making women who are struggling to breastfeed feel worse. There are plenty of things that can physically go wrong with breastfeeding, and although they can often be put right with help, the risk to a new mother is that if she thinks only a small percentage are physically incapable, then it must be *her fault* it isn't working out. Cue thinking she's a bad mother, cue stress, cue even less let-down, cue more stress, cue formula. Sound familiar?

So where does this statistic even come from? It's been bouncing around the baby world for so long that it has become an incontrovertible fact, where the source doesn't need to be cited, so its origin is a little hard to find. When I saw the Deputy Director of UNICEF's Baby Friendly Initiative in the UK quoted in an article saying 'only a very small percentage – about 1% – of women would struggle to make enough milk',[1] I wrote to ask her where the figure came from. She eventually responded, but instead of having several peer-reviewed papers sent to me, I was given links to two United Nations (UN) documents that both make blanket statements that 'virtually all women can breastfeed' without any supporting evidence. I was also given the example of a breastfeeding clinic in the UK where only 2% of mothers were deemed to have a 'pathological insufficiency' of milk, and was pointed to Norway's breastfeeding initiation rate of 99% as further proof (even though initiation is a completely separate thing from successful lactation).[2] Needless to say, none of this is robust evidence, and, frankly, I was disappointed and surprised that the UNICEF representative hadn't been able to give me more hard data to back up her statement.

However, after some digging of my own I discovered the 1% to 5% figure seems to be attributed to an American study published in 1990.[3] If you're thinking that it's odd that such an oft-quoted statistic emanated from only *one* study then you'd be right.

CASE STUDY

'I thought not being able to breastfeed meant I wasn't a good mother'

I was worried I wouldn't be able to make enough milk because of my small breast size, but every doctor I talked to said it was fine. When my daughter was born, we had a great latch, but she acted a little funny. That night she screamed, the next day she looked a little yellow in certain light, that night she wouldn't rest and felt hot and was still acting funny (feeding and then acting like she couldn't wake up), so we took her to the hospital. They kept wanting to give her a bottle (she was dehydrated and it was hard to get an IV in) but I kept refusing because of people telling me about 'booby traps' and such. It wasn't until I had seen them trying for literally hours, her sobbing for hours and losing consciousness from pain, that I prayed and felt like a bottle would only help, and I allowed it. It still took hours until they got an IV in (on her head). I continued to express or pump but I couldn't get much milk, and the exhaustion and trauma . . . I was pretty out of it.

By day six my breasts were definitely not engorging. They contacted an expert and she came and measured me. Next thing, she told me I had hypoplastic breasts with inadequate mammary tissue, and said that I was the reason formula was made.

I received almost no information when I started bottle-feeding. A lot of the doctors and nurses laughed and joked about how I should feel relieved that I was unable to nurse and didn't have to. No one addressed the loss, no one talked to us about depression, which I probably had.

I had always associated breastfeeding with being a good mom. I'm Mormon and we have very high breastfeeding rates. Every mom I babysat for had breastfed, my mom had breastfed and donated, grandma was a wet nurse. I took it as a sign I wasn't a good enough mom since every other mom breastfed and it was just a normal part of being a mom. I remember a time when I sat on the couch and sobbed for hours just holding my baby, and telling my husband that even adoptive moms can breastfeed, she deserves a better mom. He was bewildered. To him, baby was fed, happy, growing strong, it was what I had wanted for 30 years, and I was missing it sitting and crying about how I wasn't a good mom when he could see I was a great mom.

With each of my next two children I have been able to breastfeed a little more each time. But I recognise now that formula is a lifesaver. It allows us to be moms no matter the situation, and the babies turn out fine.

Emily, Colorado, USA, mother to H, 6 years old, G,
3 years old, and P, 1 year old

The other problem is that the 1990 American study has several limitations, which means its results should never have become used as the definitive measure of the ability to breastfeed.

Firstly, it wasn't even to look at that simple question of how many mothers don't produce enough milk – it was examining how breast size, shape and augmentation affected milk supply. Secondly, it looked at only 319 white, middle-class first-time American mothers who were all highly motivated to breastfeed, not a representative sample of a diverse population. Of those women, it found that 10% needed help and 5% weren't able to produce enough milk at all. If one in 20 highly motivated, well-resourced women aren't able to produce enough milk, how much higher is that figure likely to be among the wider community who don't eat as well, have more stressful life situations, and lack access to quality healthcare? We don't know, because since then there has been a lot of research into why women stop breastfeeding, but very little into 'primary lactation failure'. The third problem lies with how the study has become used. It only studied a mother's milk production, but it is often interpreted as meaning that only 5% of women can't breastfeed, and, as we know, there is so much more to successful breastfeeding than simply whether a mother has enough supply.

Why am I struggling with breastfeeding?[4]

Here are some of the most common reasons why women may struggle to produce enough milk, or may find breastfeeding physically more difficult:

- being a first-time mum
- being overweight or obese
- being an older mother
- delivering via caesarean section
- experiencing a difficult birth, especially with excessive blood loss
- experiencing fertility problems
- breast reduction surgery
- having flat or inverted nipples
- polycystic ovary syndrome (PCOS)
- hypoplasia, also known as insufficient glandular tissue or IGT (a condition where breast tissue does not develop sufficiently to produce enough milk). This is thought of as rare, but is believed to be becoming more common due to fertility treatments enabling more women who have trouble conceiving or staying pregnant to deliver healthy babies. Often, the underlying conditions behind fertility problems correspond with IGT. Women with both small and large breasts can be hypoplastic.[5]

Some of the emotional and psychological reasons why women find breastfeeding difficult or even repulsive include:

- previous eating disorders and body dysmorphia
- previous sexual assault
- being in an abusive relationship
- dysphoric milk ejection reflex or d-mer (a rare condition where lactating women experience dysphoria or negative emotions just before milk release, which then lasts for a few minutes)
- experiencing postnatal depression and anxiety (we'll talk about this more in Chapter 4 – breastfeeding can also be a positive experience for women with postnatal depression or anxiety)
- being introverted, shy or unconfident
- feeling out of control, valuing body autonomy or simply not liking it.[6]

And, of course, breastfeeding is a two-way street. It's not just what the mum does, but also what baby does, and here too we find a number of barriers to breastfeeding or digesting breast milk:

- prematurity (babies may be born prior to the suck/swallow/breath reflexes being developed)
- high palates, lip ties or tongue ties (short frenulum)
- intolerances or allergies to foods eaten by the mother and passed via breast milk, or to breast milk itself (there is emerging evidence that babies can be allergic to breast milk, despite what some websites will tell you)[7]
- jaundice or drowsiness
- reflux, including silent reflux
- low blood sugar, for example in a baby born to a diabetic mother
- certain rare metabolic diseases such as galactosaemia.

IMPORTANT NOTE: If you or your baby are currently experiencing any of these difficulties, or suspect you might be, immediately seek professional medical advice. None of these problems (except galactosaemia) means you need to stop breastfeeding, and with the right support and help you may be able to overcome them. Please go to the Resources section at the end of the book for a list of places where you can get breastfeeding support, and for further references and information on some of the breastfeeding barriers listed.

Looking at the long lists above, we can see why simply saying '5% of women can't breastfeed' is such a misrepresentation of the difficulties experienced by mums and babies. With obesity, c-sections, and the number of older first-time mums on the rise – all risk factors for trouble breastfeeding – those increasing problems alone must make that conservative figure out of date. But even if it were true that only one in 20 women can't make enough milk to feed their babies, that is already a significant number – 36,483 women in the UK[8] and 15,479 in Australia[9] every year, to be exact, going by the latest birth statistics. By way of comparison, the same percentage of 40-year-old men have erectile dysfunction,[10] but can you imagine a man struggling to get it up being dismissed by a doctor with the words 'very few [men] really can't [get erections]. That's very, very uncommon', and being told that his problem is probably down to not having enough support. (Swap a few words, and you get a quote from a fellow of the Academy of Breastfeeding Medicine to *Time Magazine*: 'very few women really can't breastfeed. That's very, very uncommon.'[11])

As breastfeeding researcher and author Dr Marianne Neifert writes: 'The bold claims made about the infallibility of lactation are not cited about any other physiologic processes. A healthcare professional would never tell a diabetic woman that "every pancreas can make insulin" or insist to a devastated infertility patient that "every woman can get pregnant".[12] So why do so many people, so many 'experts' think it's okay to just dismiss women who struggle to breastfeed as an insignificant number, and demonise what is their most readily available, nutritionally complete alternative? I honestly don't know, but I suspect it has something to do with the moralised nature of feeding, as we'll discuss in Chapter 4, and the fact that it's something only women can do.

The insignificant truth about women who can't breastfeed

Lisa Watson, the founder of bottle-feeding peer-support charity Bottle Babies, wrote this essay on what it is like to be in the 5% of women who physically can't produce enough milk for their babies. She has kindly agreed to share an edited version of it here.

'The number of women who cannot *really* breastfeed is *so* insignificant. Almost *everyone* can breastfeed. You just have to *want* to.'

Those words, spoken to me by a 'passionate' lactivist midwife as she stood over me encouraging my one-day-old baby to stay awake by placing a cold facecloth on his naked body as I desperately tried to shove another handful of breast in his screaming mouth and catch my tears on my shoulder at the same time, ran through my mind *again*.

'You just have to *want* to.'

Boy, did I want to. Beyond that – I just presumed I would. Breastfeeding, for me, was normal. It was what my mother did, what her mother did. It was my culture, what I grew up seeing, how I thought babies were fed. I didn't know anyone who bottle-fed their baby and I wasn't going to. Why would I? I had breasts and everyone knows 'breast is best' – my baby wasn't going to miss out on the best! The breastfeeding books had been devoured, the classes attended and the organisations joined. I was *so* prepared to be a breastfeeding mum. Pity someone didn't tell me not all women *can* breastfeed.

'Women who cannot *really* breastfeed.'

Yep. That's me. No – *really*. I don't *think* I can't make enough milk to adequately nourish my child. I *know* I can't. I wasn't 'booby-trapped'.

I didn't fall for the 'evil ways of the formula companies' nor am I 'uneducated', 'lazy' or any of the other things that seem to be used as an explanation by many as to why women don't breastfeed. I just can't. Physically, I can't breastfeed. It's not my fault, it's just a part of my body which doesn't work. I wear glasses to read, too. Yet I don't feel guilty that my eyes don't work the way nature intended. Did the way I fed my baby change the type of mother I was to my child? No. I was a great mother because the love I had for him didn't come from breasts or bottles, that came from my heart. Was he showing any signs of being disadvantaged by my inability to feed him from my breasts? Not that I could see. He was happy, healthy, beautiful and too smart for his own good. I couldn't be more proud. So why was I feeling so alone, so . . . insignificant?

'So insignificant.'

It made me wonder how many other women may be part of this 'insignificant' group. How many other woman had breasts who were more ornamental than practical? Were we really insignificant? No. Not really. I found out that while there isn't any really solid scientifically backed number, most healthcare professionals estimate that around 5% of woman physically cannot breastfeed. 5%. Is that really 'insignificant'?

- *12% of women are diagnosed with breast cancer.*
- *9% of children have asthma.*
- *About 5% of 40-year-old men have erection problems.*
- *Between 2% and 5% of expectant mothers develop gestational diabetes.*
- *0.1% of the world's population has Down's syndrome.*
- *Somewhere between 1.1% and 4.2% of females suffer from bulimia nervosa in their lifetime.*
- *Globally, about 1.5% of the population has autism.*
- *About 0.1% of Australia's population has HIV.*
- *Around 1% to 2% of global deaths are by suicide.*
- *0.3% of babies are born with hearing loss.*
- *In 2009, around 0.09% of the US population was hospitalised with H1N1 (swine) flu.*
- *0.03% of babies die of SIDS (Sudden Infant Death Syndrome or cot death).*
- *0.005% of women in the UK die from cervical cancer.*

Please don't tell me that the 5% of women who physically can't breastfeed is an 'insignificant' number. It is more 'significant' than HIV,

H1N1, autism, SIDS, Down's syndrome and deaths from cervical cancer and suicide put together, if you really want to look at it that way. People don't say 'most babies live so let's not discourage people by talking about SIDS'. People don't say 'only around 5% of mothers develop gestational diabetes, it's such a small number so don't worry about it' or say that they just didn't try hard enough to overcome it.

For the mother who wants to breastfeed but can't, it is usually, at the time, the most significant hardship she feels she is facing. It may not be the most significant hardship faced in the world, but in her world it is.

So next time you want to throw around 'insignificant' numbers, maybe think about how 'insignificant' you are making that mother feel.

The statistic that I think would be much more useful to spread in baby books and antenatal classes comes from a study done in 2010, which looked at 431 Californian mums from a broad social spectrum. It found that 44% still had not had their milk come in 72 hours after birth. Consider that – nearly half of all first-time mums waited more than three days to lactate. The authors called it an 'alarmingly common problem', and if you have been in that same situation you will know how frightening it can be – a crying baby, an exhausted mum and no explanation about why you are still not producing milk.[13] And why does this matter, other than for the obvious reasons of a baby's weight loss and stress to the mother? Because mums who have breastfeeding concerns at day three are the ones who are likely to have given up breastfeeding by two months.[14]

CASE STUDY

'Bodily autonomy is a huge thing to me'

I am 37 years old and a survivor of sexual assault. Breastfeeding would have triggered memories I did not wish to revisit, so I knew that in order to be the healthiest mother possible for my child, I needed to bottle-feed her. Bodily autonomy is a huge thing to me, and retaining control over choices involving my body. I felt that bottle-feeding allowed me to have more choices and also retain ownership of my body after my baby inhabited it for nine months. I felt invaded while I was pregnant.

I think there are many women who feel this way but are too embarrassed to speak up. Rape is a sensitive subject anyway, and to admit that you can't do 'what is best' for your child really does a mental number on some women. There is such pressure that 'breast is best', but what about the mother? What about what is best for her mental health?

People will always judge you. If it's not breast versus bottle, then it's something else. I feel I have been 60% judged and 40% supported. I have been told I am a horrible person, I feed my child dog food and that I am very selfish. But the only standard I hold myself to is the health and happiness of my child. And she is ridiculously healthy, happy, gorgeous, hitting all her milestones and then some, and I am a happy, healthy mom who can relax and enjoy her child.

One of my friends saw me upset after a woman made the dog food comment to me, and said, 'Don't worry about them. They are as inconsequential as radishes.' So now I imagine a bunch of talking radishes when people make crazy comments or judgements!

Kimberly, Hiroshima, Japan, mother to Madeline, 2 years

Concerns over milk production: environmental factors

Studies consistently show that the top reasons why women stop breastfeeding are feeding difficulties and worries about their baby not getting enough milk,[15] yet these concerns are routinely dismissed by health professionals. Some of the nastier zealots accuse women of lying, of not trying hard enough – this nasty phrase will likely be familiar to too many of you.

The good news is that sensible breastfeeding advocates are recognising that women's concerns over breastfeeding difficulties and supply need to be taken seriously, and that damage is caused by the disconnect between the rhetoric that nearly every woman can breastfeed and the lived reality of so many of us. One of these advocates is Dr Alison Stuebe, a much-decorated breastfeeding researcher, physician and fellow of the

American Academy of Breastfeeding Medicine, who wrote a thoughtful blog on the question of 'How often does breastfeeding just not work?'

It is, she writes, 'a difficult [question] to answer … We also need to step back from assertions that every mother can breastfeed if she just tries hard enough. Lactation is part of normal human physiology, and like all other human physiology, it can fail. It's time to stop bickering about whether this mom tried as hard as that mom to breastfeed.'

Part of the problem in figuring out why so many women find breastfeeding challenging, Dr Stuebe writes, is because it's difficult to separate the purely physical problems from cultural, social and institutional ones.

'We're also finding that it's quite difficult to tease out the issue of "a supportive environment" versus biological problems with lactation … From a health and well-being perspective, however, I'm not sure that it matters whether we "count" both "biological" and "perceived" insufficient lactation together. The total burden of this problem is enormous, and mothers are suffering, whether they lack glandular tissue or they lack self-sufficiency and support.'[16]

Dr Stuebe hits the nail on the head when she points out that the lines between physical problems and environmental barriers are blurred. What is not in doubt though, and is worthy of much more research, is that the way we live our modern, Western lives influences our bodies' breastfeeding capabilities.

We only need to compare the Californian study mentioned above, which found that more than 44% of first-time mothers still hadn't had their milk come in by day three, with the results of studies in other, less developed countries. One, conducted in Peru, found that only 17% of first-time mothers waited until day three for their milk to arrive.[17] Another, in rural Ghana, found that less than 5% of new mothers waited that long.[18] The American mothers weren't lying about not having milk – researchers observed it actually still had not come in by day three. So why the difference? Certainly, there were disparities in age, wealth and education between the American, Peruvian and Ghanaian groups, but the fundamental biology is pretty much the same. Why then is it common for American mothers to have their milk come in late, but rare for Ghanaian mothers?

'A supportive environment'

At least part of the reason is down to our different breastfeeding environments.

We live in a weird world. On the one hand, as Western women we are told that, at all costs, the one thing we must do for our babies is breastfeed them. On the other hand, so many aspects of our modern life make it so hard: breastfeeding in public is still frequently derided, overstretched midwives often don't have time to help get it right, we don't have the widespread social support that can be needed to establish breastfeeding, we sometimes don't have enough maternity leave to enable us to meet the six-month exclusive breastfeeding goal – the list goes on, and on, and on.[19] There has been so much written on this topic it's impossible to do it justice here, but I think it's worth briefly talking about the huge problem of the lack of real-life breastfeeding role models and support systems, and the potential impact this has on our ability to nurse.

When I gave birth, I had probably seen about five people breastfeed in my entire life, and never in public. It's not that it was frowned upon, it just wasn't something I ever encountered. My mother had to go back to work when I was six weeks old, so I was moved on to formula, and even though she breastfed my two sisters, the last time she unclipped a nursing bra was 30 years ago, so she didn't have much advice. What's more, at the time I gave birth, she lived in Australia and I lived in London. She wonderfully came over to visit for the first three weeks of my baby's life, but after that she had to go back home to the other side of the world. None of my close friends had babies, and although my mothers' group and I met up once a week, we weren't hanging out in each other's houses for hours on end, helping get the hang of this feeding thing. Basically, I was alone.

Breastfeeding, although a natural bodily function, is still a learned behaviour. Back in the day, that learning would have come via our mothers, sisters and friends, not classes, books and lactation consultants. It would have been ongoing, and free. And we would have seen plenty of women breastfeeding in action before we gave birth to our own babies, so it would have seemed like a regular part of life. After a couple of generations of bottles being the preferred feeding method of the majority, the collective memory of breastfeeding as the norm has faded. The breastfeeding advocate and scholar Berenice Hausman argues: 'Once a culture loses its common memory of breastfeeding by only one or two generations of mothers, bottle-feeding becomes not only normative, but the paradigm from which accepted ideas about maternity, infancy, and development emerge.'[20]

I agree with her, but I think she gives only half of the picture. Competing with the normative nature of bottle-feeding is the equally strong message that has been spread so successfully by the medical community, governments and social groups: that good mothers breastfeed, and bad mothers bottle-feed. As women, we find ourselves caught in the middle of the two messages – bottles are normal but bad; breastfeeding is less normal in some communities but good.[21] (And there are also social circles where breastfeeding is normal and bottle-feeding is odd.) On the one hand, society still makes it hard for us to breastfeed; on the other, society tells us we must. Awesome.

Your own struggles to breastfeed have probably been fuelled not only by physical inability (and certainly not by a simple lack of will) but by a society that pays lip service to breastfeeding but doesn't support it.

The Himba

For a little detour that might help highlight how non-breastfeeding friendly our own environments are, let me take you to the deserts of Namibia. There, we meet the Himba, a tribe of semi-nomadic pastoralists whose way of life hasn't changed much in centuries – they still live in mud huts, tend their goat herds, and the women wear traditional dress that doesn't cover their breasts. They are a living, breathing vestige of a traditional tribal society, enduring in the twenty-first century.

Pretty much 100% of all Himba mothers breastfeed, and do so exclusively for a number of months. If there were any society where the statement 'very few women can't breastfeed' would ring true, it would be here. But there are a number of key differences between the Himba's lives and our own, and having no cars and no internet and covering themselves in red ochre for decoration is just the beginning. Dr Brooke Scelza, a behavioural ecologist (a type of anthropologist) from UCLA in California has studied the Himba and their breastfeeding patterns.

She's also mother to a nine-month-old baby, so has a pretty sharp view on how their culture compares with our modern, Western lives.

'It's a very different situation for sure,' she told me one Sunday night over the phone from Los Angeles, after handing over her own baby to her husband for bed time. The key difference with the Himba, she says, is that expectant mothers move back to their own mothers' compounds when they are ready to give birth, and stay there for up to a year afterwards.

'Their mothers seem to be really key in terms of early learning about breastfeeding and actual support,' she says. 'Their mother actually shows them . . . how to put the baby to the breast, how to latch on.' Also, because grandmother, mother and baby all tend to sleep in the same hut, the grandmother helps the mother in the middle of the night. Just like having your own maternity nurse, but free! What I would have given for one of those!

'This visitation practice is pretty key to basically giving them 24-hour support for the first few months,' says Dr Scelza. 'This is critical for a number of reasons, not just because they have somebody there to help them do things like wake up and feed the baby, but I think that being back home with their families reduces their workload too. So just having that generalised support means they can spend a lot more time doing nothing but caring for their babies, which is quite different from my context where I had to go back to work after five weeks and my family was far away.' She pauses, and then sighs: 'We're just much more detached from our extended families in the West.'[22]

The lives of Himba women and our own could not be more different, yet we are expected to physiologically perform in the same way after our babies are born. We are managing careers, other children, bills and households all on our own. Himba women have 24-hour support from their own mothers and extended family, reduced workloads, and none of the stress of trying to maintain monetary income to pay for modern lives. No wonder they get the hang of breastfeeding and so many of us struggle. (By the way, the Himba also often start supplementing with fermented goat's milk when their baby is as young as three months. Dr Scelza is still investigating why, but some of the women she interviewed mentioned concerns over supply. It seems even a people who are the most successful breastfeeders in the world wouldn't meet the international goals for exclusive breastfeeding duration, and that failure has nothing to do with the influence of formula.)

The enormous differences between the Himba and ourselves show the futility in a modern world of inferring that because breastfeeding is 'natural' we all should be able to do it as easily as our tribal ancestors. It overplays the biological and ignores the social – humans 'naturally' group in families and villages for survival. That makes our modern living arrangements, separated from parents and siblings, in apartments or houses where we can't turn to our neighbour for support, thoroughly unnatural in terms of social evolution. What's more, Himba women have extra help from their families for up to a year, and may even work less during that time because their extended family can help to support them. In Britain, according to the law, women are entitled to take up to a year of maternity leave, but only the first six weeks are mandated to be at 90% of their full pay; after that, it's a bare minimum.[23] In Australia, parents can take a year's parental leave but there is no mandated minimum pay.[24] When having a baby means potentially paying a severe financial penalty, that's not protecting a mother–baby relationship. So why should we expect our bodies to behave in a 'natural' way when the rest of our lives are no longer structured 'naturally'?

It's a point that Dr Katie Hinde, who runs the Comparative Lactation Laboratory at Harvard University, agrees with. As a researcher who spends her life studying the milk of primates, including humans, she's a big supporter of breastfeeding, but she also has a wonderfully pragmatic view about its demands, and how incompatible they often are with our modern lives. She has also spent time with the Himba, and has seen how important social support is to their breastfeeding success.

'The "natural" condition for humans is to have a support network that helps with your problems,' she told me from Boston. 'The difficulty comes with the myth that just because something is natural means it's easy. They aren't the same thing. Walking on two legs is what humans do, yet we all know that everybody starts out being pretty bad at it. The idea that natural means easy is a myth that is very damaging to women.'[25]

As a society, we have come some way in trying to make up for this loss of social support for breastfeeding with antenatal classes, breastfeeding groups, baby cafes, breastfeeding hotlines and the advent of professional lactation consultants. These are all important and can make a big difference to women learning to breastfeed. They are nearly all achievements of the breastfeeding lobby and dedicated lactivists, and we should be grateful for the work and pressure that brought these changes about. But they aren't complete solutions to the challenges of breastfeeding in the modern world: breastfeeding groups can be a wonderful support but there has to be one in your area and you have to leave your house, baby in tow, to get to one; breastfeeding hotlines can help rectify some issues, but if you need hands-on support they can fall short; and lactation consultants can give that hands-on support, but usually only if you have the means to pay for it. What women are told and taught about breastfeeding before the baby arrives is particularly problematic.

'Pressure over not breastfeeding gave me PTSD'

CASE STUDY

As I type, I'm breastfeeding Aidan, my eight-week-old son. Two years ago, I breastfed Rory for 20 days, before giving up completely because of severe pain. I was relieved to stop when I did, and recovered well to enjoy most of my first six months of motherhood. However, there were occasions when I felt judged by friends and strangers. For example, I joined a postnatal yoga class and dropped out after a few weeks when the yoga teacher kept relating individual poses to the physicality of breastfeeding – despite knowing that I was the only mum in the class who was exclusively bottle-feeding her baby.

I started to feel angry about being quizzed by opinionated people – many of the women felt free to tell me how 'lucky' they felt to have found breastfeeding 'easy'. I developed an aversion to reading the packaging of my formula milk. It felt like being forced to read daily reminders of my 'failure'. I researched the desktop evidence and although there was plenty of rational reassurance that formula milk doesn't harm your baby, I felt devastated by some of the more outlandish claims made about my son's long-term prospects, and the depth of the bond we'd formed. It triggered a deep, long-lasting anxiety and I was diagnosed with post-traumatic stress disorder when Rory was 10 months old.

continued

continued from previous page

And then my 'luck' changed. My GP referred me to an excellent therapist, who helped to address the traumatic memories triggering my anger and anxiety. Going back to full-time work helped me to close the door on the bitterness I felt.

When I contemplated having my second child, I considered using bottles straight away. My family were keen for me to give some colostrum and I decided to try again. This time, I negotiated better postnatal care and feeding support. I also pushed back on official pressure by insisting that the 'breast is best' posters in my antenatal consultation room were taken down during my appointments. (The midwives were surprisingly sympathetic.) I felt quite neutral about how my baby would be fed, as I realise that formula gives me a solid back-up plan. With Aidan, I've taken it each feed at a time. And I don't have any worries that one son has had a better start. Both are healthy, beautiful boys and they are growing at a rate of knots. I am a very proud – and yes, lucky – mama!

Annabel, London, mother to Rory, 2, and Aidan, 8 weeks

'No one tells you': the realities of breastfeeding

How often have you sat with a new mum and heard her say, 'No one told me it would be this hard'? How often has that new mum been you?

A common theme from research from around the world into how we feed our babies is that the lack of realistic expectations around breastfeeding is setting women up to fail.[26] This will likely come as no surprise to you. It certainly doesn't to me. I've forgotten exactly what went on in my two-hour breastfeeding class prior to my daughter being born (except for the video of a half-naked postnatal woman with ENORMOUS breasts smiling maniacally as she hand-expressed into a saucer – try as I might I can't get that image out of my brain). However, I do know that at no stage did my instructor say, 'Even if you're doing it right it could still hurt for weeks,' or 'Sometimes you'll be so tired you'll forget your own name,' or 'There's this thing called "cluster feeding" where you won't get off the couch between 6 and 10 p.m., so forget about having any time alone with your husband.' Those would all have been really helpful things to know. They wouldn't have changed my decision to breastfeed but they would definitely have saved me a few tears of frustration.

Sasha says:

It seems unclear whose job it is to tell pregnant women about infant feeding. My own experience was a single two-hour session with the NCT class, which was optional, paid for (and pretty expensive at that) and mostly unhelpful. For the large proportion of mums-to-be who don't opt for additional NCT classes, it doesn't seem to be mentioned during antenatal care very much at all. This clearly needs addressing, as we discuss below.

The evidence is actually mixed about the extent to which antenatal breastfeeding education improves initiation, duration and exclusivity,[27] but the health community finally seems to be coming to the realisation that maybe the results have something to do with the quality of the education. Scottish research into infant feeding experiences published in 2012, gathered from a series of in-depth interviews with 72 mothers and their family members, found the biggest problem for new mums was a 'clash between overt or covert infant feeding idealism and the reality experienced'.[28] Mothers they spoke to described feeding education as 'unrealistic, overly technical and rules-based', which, in turn, 'undermine[d] women's confidence'. In another study into the physical challenges of early breastfeeding, Canadian and American women repeatedly described being surprised by the pain and physical demands of breastfeeding. The common theme was 'no one tells you' what it will be like. And the pain had consequences – some women said it was so bad it impacted on their relationship with their baby.[29] If they were warned about that possible pain, would they have felt less resentment? Maybe.

NCT, Britain's largest non-government provider of antenatal classes, did an impact review of its education in 2013 and found that a key issue was that 'Mothers who run into breastfeeding problems sometimes feel that they have been given unrealistic expectations in antenatal classes.' You don't say? Those videos of women smiling beatifically as they feed and the unhurried, non-breast-squeezing midwife don't mimic reality? No way! In a very welcome recognition of its own shortcomings, the charity found it needed to 'shift the focus from seeking to influence initial feeding decisions towards supporting mothers and fathers over many months', as well as to 'promote the idea that there is a necessary "adjustment and investment period" during the early weeks after birth in order for breastfeeding to be established'.[30] To put that in another way, they need to spend less time lecturing women about why they must breastfeed, and spend more time telling them what it might actually be like. Sounds pretty sensible to me.

Antenatal educators must know they run the risk of scaring the bejeezus out of new mums if they're honest about how hard breastfeeding can be. And they have a point. Women who feel more confident about their ability to breastfeed *before* they have a baby tend to feed for longer. Maybe this is why 'no one tells you' what it's like, because they're worried that if you knew it was possible for your nipple to be so gnawed off that it is actually hanging from your breast by a scrap of skin (yes, it is!) then you'd be more ready to give up, and too scared to try in the first place. But this paternalistic approach hectors women into feeling they must follow a particular path, and then leaves them without the coping tools when the shit hits the fan, and that's not fair.

Sasha says:

Additionally, by demonising formula milk and giving mums the message that even the smallest amount of formula will ruin their perfect, breastfed infant, we are excluding the option of formula top-ups while milk supply is being established. As you will see in the next chapter, this can be an effective strategy for mums with delayed lactation for improving the overall length of breastfeeding.

When I asked Dr Katie Hinde of Harvard University what she would like to see change in the way we approach infant feeding, she came back with three suggestions. Bear in mind that these come from a woman who spends her life studying the breast milk of various mammals, including humans, and thinks that it is amazing. I'll quote her at length because her suggestions are so sensible:

> 66 One, I would like discussions of breastfeeding to happen in a nuanced way, during prenatal care. Women are prepared for the pain of childbirth and they still go ahead and do it, and I think we should prepare them for the challenges of

breastfeeding . . . before difficulties happen, because once
difficulties happen they can be harder to correct than if you had
just prevented them in the first place.

Two, I would like to see a much better discussion of the
institutional obstacles that make it so much more difficult for
mothers to breastfeed. Maternity leave, time to establish mother–
infant bonds to stimulate milk production. A clean and safe place
for you to pump at work, or ways for babies to come and visit
you at work . . . More acceptance of public breastfeeding. We
need to improve institutional and societal infrastructure to make
breastfeeding a more viable option for more women.

And the third thing is that we need to have a much better
conversation about not demonising women who do not
breastfeed. There are these societal and institutional difficulties
and there are these issues with supply, and supplementing or
replacing breast milk with formula may be holistically the best
decision for that particular baby and that family at that time.
And I think we need to have a lot more respect for the many
many challenges of breastfeeding . . . We're doing a disservice
to moms by saying you can only be a good mom if you follow a
certain set of paths and you can't deviate from that. And I don't
think this is fair. It's a complex thing. Is breastfeeding oftentimes
healthiest for mothers and infants? Yes. Does healthiest always
mean best? Not necessarily.[31]

I have never before wanted to hug someone I've only met over Skype,
but if I could have leaned through my computer and given Katie Hinde
a big bear squeeze I would have. Hallelujah! A breast milk researcher
who realises that there are women attached to those breasts, who have
feelings and needs and aren't just jugs of 'liquid gold', one who *believes*
that mothers have legitimate issues with supply and aren't lying when
they say they don't produce enough, and who accepts that sometimes
formula may be the better option for a family.

Sometimes support isn't enough

Lactivists typically agree with Katie's second, well-made, point,
ignoring the first and definitely the third. The standard response of

Sasha says:

As a paediatrician, I had received comprehensive education about the practicalities of breastfeeding from midwives and neonatal nurses, had helped numerous new mums to 'get a good latch', and had assessed babies and new mums from every aspect of the spectrum for breastfeeding technique.

But still, when it came to my own first experience of breastfeeding, I felt utterly bewildered. It hurt so much, not for hours or days but for weeks. My bleeding, cracked nipples needed to heal, not be split open again by each two-hourly feed. I seemed to never have enough milk, and chased my tail round an endless circle of feeding, expressing, EBM (expressed breast milk) bottle top-ups and feeding again. A posterior tongue tie seemed minor to my doctor eyes, but felt hugely significant to my mother eyes. I was so disappointed in myself; I had imagined myself a happy, natural breastfeeder with my years of experience and bags of commitment to breastfeeding. But instead I resented it, dreaded it and ended up partly hating it. Not the bit where I held my beautiful daughter in my arms and fed her from my own body. But the parts before and after when I couldn't put a towel round myself after the shower for months because my nipples were too sore, or the extra 30 minutes of precious sleep lost in the middle of countless nights when I was pumping after my baby went to sleep post-feed, not lying down beside her.

I managed four and a half months of exclusive breastfeeding, although many feeds were given as EBM via bottle to give my poor boobs a break. I was proud of myself for not giving any formula until that point. But since then I have asked myself many times 'Was it worth it?' I remember times when I left my daughter crying just to get a few more minutes of pumping time to get enough milk for her next feed. With all I have learned from the evidence and literature surrounding the benefits of breastfeeding, I do not think I would put myself, or my baby, through that again. I would try to breastfeed and I would do so exclusively if it works for my baby and me next time. But if it doesn't, I would feel happy to reach for the formula in the knowledge that it is a balanced, informed choice I am making and that formula and a sane mother might just be a far better combination than breast and an exhausted, slightly mad, resentful one. It seems a pretty sensible choice to me, both as a mum and as a doctor.

the breastfeeding lobby as to why so many women struggle is lack of support. A typical lactivist reply is: 'The only reason breastfeeding is seen as so much harder is because our culture and often our medical professionals totally undermine it.'[32] While support is clearly a huge part of getting breastfeeding right, as the Himba showed us, the fact is, sometimes you can have all the support in the world and it just doesn't work.

In chatting with Dr Mandy Belfort, the lead author of a 2013 Harvard study that associated improved intelligence with breastfeeding (and another very sensible and balanced breast milk researcher), she happened to mention that she had a few fellow paediatrician friends who had struggled to breastfeed. '[They] found after their children were born that they just weren't able to produce enough milk despite enormous amounts of support. They just couldn't do it. Their bodies just didn't make the milk and they went through that grieving and feeling of guilt but ultimately they recognised that not feeding their baby formula was going to be harmful.'[33]

Dr Belfort's friends aren't that unusual. One small survey of medical professionals with young families, all women who were highly motivated to breastfeed, found that two-thirds had problems, and of those women, a quarter never resolved them.[34] The paediatrician who looked after me and my sisters when we were growing up told me that in his career he had seen more than a dozen babies of doctors, nurses and breastfeeding counsellors who were severely underweight because breastfeeding wasn't working, but the mothers refused to see it. Support clearly wasn't the issue for these women.

Is the modern world affecting our breast milk?

All of this makes me wonder if the constant refrain of women 'just needing more support' isn't a cop-out.[35] While at least not putting blame on individual women for being lazy or not committed, the support argument still implies that 'nearly every woman can breastfeed'. But what if, in our modern society, that is no longer true? There is emerging evidence that everyday chemicals are disrupting our endocrine (hormonal) system, the same system that is involved in breast milk production.[36] What if, say, our prolific technology use is affecting our ability to breastfeed? Or the separation from our extended families affects our emotions, which then affects our let-down? I don't know whether this is the case, but surely they are possibilities worth exploring?

So, to Katie Hinde's excellent list of what she would change in approaches to infant feeding, I would like to add one more suggestion: I would like to see much more recognition by clinicians that when women say they're having trouble breastfeeding they're not lying, and it's not that they just haven't tried hard enough. How about we shift some of those research pounds from yet another study into breastfeeding and IQ and into looking at why it is that women in the developed world experience more delays in having their milk come in than women in Africa. Or into how smartphone use might affect let-down. Or into finding out *exactly* what proportion of women don't produce milk, rather than just trotting out a 24-year-old statistic from a study that wasn't even into generalised milk production problems anyway. All of these things might not only help a lot of women feel it's OK that they are not breastfeeding, it might actually turn up some ways to help combat those challenges to improve breastfeeding rates. Because, let's face it, the status quo of pressure and guilt isn't working.

A call for personalised breastfeeding goals

With all of this in mind, perhaps it's time to re-examine the breastfeeding goals we all receive by default when we get pregnant: six months exclusive, and one or more years in combination with other foods. Research consistently finds that a majority of Western women aren't reaching their breastfeeding goals.[37] That is typically taken as evidence that we need more support for breastfeeding, which is undeniably true. But what if, in addition to that, the goals themselves are unrealistic in the first place? If a 22-year-old woman living in an inner-city deprived area, who comes from two generations of bottle-feeders, is given the same breastfeeding goal of six months as a 35-year-old university-educated woman who was breastfed herself as a baby, it's like saying they should both be able to climb a mountain, and then giving Lady A Mount Everest and Lady B Primrose Hill. (Research shows that successful breastfeeders tend to be older, wealthier and more educated and were breastfed themselves.) I'm not saying Lady A can't surmount that peak, but it's hardly doling out an equal challenge.

The authors of the 2012 Scottish study that found that many women believed breastfeeding education to be unrealistic, and ultimately undermined their confidence, came to the conclusion that the international six-month exclusive breastfeeding goal was 'unhelpful' for individual women.[38] That's a pretty radical statement from a bunch of health researchers, but it reflects the reality felt by many women rather than the aspiration of many health workers and politicians.

Perhaps it's time to re-evaluate, recognising that the broad-brush targets for breastfeeding are not significantly closer to being met than they were 20 years ago, and adjust our expectations accordingly. I would argue that these expectations need to be adjusted on an *individual* level – a personalised breastfeeding plan, if you will.

Imagine if a woman, before she gave birth, could sit down with a one-on-one feeding educator, talk about her personal circumstances, and then figure out what might be achievable. For a woman who had already breastfed one baby, didn't have to go back to work for a year and was healthy and active, perhaps six months exclusive and then however long she felt like it, in combination with other foods, is an achievable target. For an overweight woman who had trouble conceiving, perhaps a more appropriate plan might be to start breastfeeding with added syringed top-ups of formula or donated breast milk for a month while her supply built, and then reassess. For a busy mother of three with her own business, perhaps a target of six weeks exclusive breastfeeding, and then five months of mixed feeding, might be an achievable goal.

Women, especially second-time mums, do this informally, but while we're all still being bound to the official target of six months, in the eyes of the health sector the vast majority of us are failures. That's not good for mothers on a personal level, nor for society on a broader level.

Sasha says:

We all sit down with our midwife or other healthcare professional in mid to late pregnancy and form a birth plan of what particular, personal choices we would like to make about the place and manner of our labour and delivery. Why is it any different to do the same with a breastfeeding counsellor and make some sensible, realistic and informed decisions about infant feeding?

The fight must continue for better support of breastfeeding: more realistic education, better midwife and health visitor care, freely available lactation consultants, better maternity provisions, more acceptance of public nursing, and protection of the right to nurse and pump at work. But we need to begin a new fight – one that seeks to give women and their needs, capabilities and complex lives equal footing in the baby feeding relationship. We need to trust that mothers want to do what's best for their baby, and that 'what's best' is part of a hugely complex web of decisions involving not only mother and baby, but a family, a community and society as a whole.

We bottle-feed for a number of reasons. Those reasons should be respected, not derided. Mothers who bottle-feed should be afforded that same respect.

CASE STUDY

'I chose to bottle-feed from birth'

While most mothers want to breastfeed and end up using a bottle earlier than they had planned, some women choose to bottle-feed from birth. It goes without saying that this is an equally valid choice for mothers to make. Mary's story shows how you can raise a happy, healthy, bonded baby who was bottle-fed from the outset.

I fully support breastfeeding, but strongly believe it's a personal choice. When I was pregnant with my son Harvey, the thought of a baby sucking on my nipple made my skin crawl. Also, having suffered with some depression in the past, I didn't want to feel trapped by the baby as I had seen happen to some of my friends, and I wanted to also be able to share everything with my husband who wanted to be very hands-on. Many people said I should have expressed my milk but 'I'm not a cow' went through my head several times!

Towards the end of my pregnancy I was pleasantly surprised by how accepted it was by midwives. We went to a 'parent craft class' and out of the 15 couples we were the only ones who honestly and openly said we planned to bottle-feed. The midwife who ran the group praised us for being honest and said she would rather people didn't just say what they thought midwives wanted to hear. She said midwives spend a lot of time helping people to breastfeed who as soon as they go home just bottle-feed anyway because they think they will be judged in hospital.

I felt quite good about that but she said she couldn't give us any advice on bottle-feeding as they weren't allowed to promote it.* I didn't get any judgement in hospital, which I was quite surprised about. The judgement only came when we went to local baby groups, from breastfeeding mums. They said they couldn't understand why I didn't even try. I did notice, however, that the majority of those babies seemed to be feeding almost constantly and had very tired mummies who seemed slightly envious of my chilled-out baby who fed every four hours like clockwork.

My now 2½-year-old son has not had any more illnesses or issues than the exclusively breastfed babies the same age as him, and certainly doesn't have any attachment issues. I felt no issues with bonding and very much enjoyed our feeding time snuggles. I am happy and confident in how we fed our son and it worked well for us as a family. It's not taking the 'easy way out', as some have said.

Breastfeeding is not for everyone and it breaks my heart to see people who beat themselves up and feel so bad about themselves for not doing it and feel like failures. If women didn't feel so pressured, I strongly believe postnatal depression rates would drop.

Mary, Sussex, mother to Harvey, 2½, with baby number two on the way

* This is actually incorrect and a misinterpretation of health guidelines. If parents request information on bottle-feeding before the birth, they are supposed to be given verbal advice and instruction, though not a demonstration. We go into this more in Chapter 4.

2 Why bottle-feeding will not make your baby fat, sick or stupid

'Breast is best' has to be one of the catchiest marketing slogans ever. It's short, it's pithy, it rhymes. It's certainly a lot easier to remember than, 'breast milk is better than formula, but some of its touted benefits probably come from the act of breastfeeding, as well as simply the type of parenting provided by mothers who choose to breastfeed, and formula is also a nutritionally complete way to feed your baby, so don't sweat it too much'.

But while my revised slogan won't be making it onto a poster anytime soon, that is exactly what we want to show you in this chapter.

We'll start by giving you a primer in how breastfeeding research is conducted, showing you its pitfalls and the X factor that affects results. Then we'll go on to show you the Truth Gap – how what we're told about the benefits of breastfeeding isn't mirrored by the research. Finally, we'll delve into the research itself to demonstrate in detail why, despite breast milk being great stuff and ounce-for-ounce better than formula, it is not a magic elixir.

The problem with breastfeeding studies

Here's a quick reminder of what we're commonly told the scientifically proven benefits of breastfeeding are: it helps prevent obesity, diabetes, diarrhoea, vomiting, coughs, colds, ear infections, sudden infant death syndrome (SIDS), eczema, allergies and some cancers in children. For mums, the list is smaller but no less appealing: it reduces the risk of ovarian and breast cancers, acts as a natural contraceptive, and gets you back to your pre-pregnancy weight faster. And don't forget the all-important bond it is supposed to create between mother and child.

We'll break down some of that list in a moment, but before we go on, there's a key point you need to know about virtually all breastfeeding research: it doesn't, and can't, compare like for like when it comes to studying children who are bottle-fed as opposed to breastfed.

To get a true comparison, scientists would take a large number of mothers and their babies, and randomly put them into two groups: one group would be told to use only formula and the other would be told to only breastfeed. The random allocation would ensure that in each group there was an equal distribution of mothers with characteristics that affect their children's health outcomes – things like smoking and drinking status of the mothers, their intelligence, education levels, race, class and marital status. It would also give an equal distribution of other factors that influence children but are much more difficult for scientists to measure – kindness, the ability to show affection, patience, enthusiasm for motherhood, optimism, the mother's happiness with her relationship with her partner and her general outlook on life.

Because this split creates two groups that are as equal as possible in the maternal physical, mental and emotional characteristics that influence children's outcomes, it would allow researchers to get a true measure of the difference in the health of babies in each of the groups. These differences would then be explained by the only remaining differentiating factor – whether they were breastfed or bottle-fed.

This is called a randomised controlled trial, and it is the gold standard for research.

Observational research

Except, that's not how breastfeeding studies are conducted. Because breast milk has been accepted as the superior food source for decades, it is deemed to be unethical to force a woman to bottle-feed in the name of medical research.

Instead, breastfeeding science is based on *observational* studies, where babies whose mothers have *already chosen* to breastfeed are examined and compared with babies whose mothers have chosen to exclusively bottle-feed or combination feed. The outcomes are then observed and conclusions drawn from them.

This may seem like splitting statisticians' hairs, but it is actually crucially important, because women who *choose* to breastfeed are, in general, different from women who choose to bottle-feed. For starters, women who begin and continue to breastfeed are more likely to be older, work in managerial or professional occupations, and have had a tertiary education, all factors that improve a child's health and academic outcomes.[1] Some breastfeeding studies, especially more recent ones, try to make up for these variables that are likely to skew results (known as 'confounders' in the statistics business) by adjusting the results to negate their effect. But there is a myriad of possible confounders in any research that looks at the health and social outcomes of children, including education, social class, single parenting and even smoking status. Older research papers generally don't take all, and sometimes not even many, of these confounders into account.

Jargon buster: 'confounder'

In statistics, a confounder, or a confounding variable, is an extra related factor that masks the true relationship between A and B, when the question 'How does A affect B?' is asked. For example, if I were studying whether heavy metal music makes people deaf, I might see that more heavy metal fans go deaf than the average population. From that I might conclude that there is something about heavy metal music itself that makes people deaf. However, of course, the confounding variable in this case is the volume at which people listen to heavy metal. It's not the *music* that makes people deaf, it's the *volume* of the music – any type of loud music would be just as likely to make people deaf, but heavy metal fans tend to turn the music up more loudly than classical fans. Unless I account for the volume of their headphones, I won't have a true reflection of the relationship between heavy metal and deafness.

If statisticians know that a particular confounder exists, they are able to adjust the results accordingly so that the effect of the confounder is minimised or eliminated. So, for example, because we know that a mother's IQ influences her child's IQ, any study into the relationship between breastfeeding and intelligence needs to account for the influence of the mother's IQ (and for other confounders) so that any results reflect only the relationship between the feeding method and intelligence, and not the other factors. Statisticians have ways of doing this, but they have to know that the confounder exists in the first place.

The decision to breastfeed – the X factor in scientific research

What's more, academic research can't factor out the effect of what could be the most basic confounder of all – the *decision* to breastfeed. A much-quoted study of mothers and babies in the Scottish city of Dundee found that mums who chose to bottle-feed from birth were more likely to be unhappy about being pregnant, skip antenatal appointments, and not bother to go to parenting classes. In general, they were less dedicated to being the best mothers they could be.[2] Conversely, women who choose to breastfeed from birth, and who keep it up through all the difficulties, are probably more committed to doing the best they can for their baby.

Before you throw this book away in disgust, I'm not saying that you're not committed to being a good mother if you choose not to breastfeed, or if you started but it didn't work out – I want to show that the very opposite is true. Very many bottle-feeding parents (and certainly *all* who I have met) are very committed to their children's health, but have chosen or been forced to bottle-feed for a wide variety of reasons. They express their commitment to the health of their children in other ways, such as by preparing healthy meals, keeping their child's toys and play area supremely clean, or reading to and spending quality time with their children.

However, researchers have recognised that in a world where the 'breast is best' message has been internalised by all women, starting and continuing to breastfeed in spite of difficulties can be an indicator of mothers who will go the extra mile for their kids. The effects of that commitment cascade down through every aspect of a child's life, and cannot be adequately statistically accounted for when studying the effects of breast milk.

In her meticulously researched book *Is Breast Best?: Taking on the Breastfeeding Experts and the New High Stakes of Motherhood*, the American academic Joan B. Wolf suggests that 'breastfeeding cannot be clearly distinguished from the decision to breastfeed; the choice to initiate and continue breastfeeding might signal a variety of health-promoting behaviours on the part of the child's caretakers, and the decision to breastfeed could represent an approach to child care that is far more important than breastfeeding itself'.[3]

In other words, a woman who is supremely committed to keeping her baby healthy is more likely to choose to breastfeed because she has read all about its touted benefits. But she is also probably more likely to ask people to wash their hands before they pick up her baby, to keep her rugged up if she has a cold, and to talk to her a lot, all factors that promote health and intelligence. So when that child has fewer colds than the kids in her class, or does better in exams, what was it that made the difference? Was it the breast milk, or was it those other, extra, immeasurable things – the X factor?

In truth, scientists themselves don't know, and many of the more recent and thorough studies acknowledge this. As a major review of breastfeeding studies commissioned by the US Department of Health and Human Services (known as the AHRQ report) explicitly states: 'Although it is possible to control for differences in demographic factors, it may not be possible to control for behaviour intrinsic in the desire to breastfeed.'[4]

It is a fact that children who were breastfed as babies are generally healthier than those who were bottle-fed. The breast milk itself is certainly one of the reasons for this; however, there is a whole host of other complex influences that affect health outcomes for children, including the mother's commitment to her baby's health, and these are downplayed when we are simply told that 'breast is best'.

The Truth Gap: what we're told the research says, and what it actually says

There are literally more than a thousand studies published every year on breastfeeding and breast milk. Big studies, small studies – scientists love looking at the stuff.

Most of these studies are published in journals for which you need a special subscription to get access, so us mere non-medically trained mortals rely on doctors, midwives, science journalists and plenty of internet forums to read, distil and serve up the information in an easily digestible form. When we're told, 'studies show', or 'research has found', we trust that we're being given an easy-to-understand approximation of the science, which we can then apply to our lives.

However, the odd thing about breastfeeding research that you wouldn't pick up unless you actually read the original studies yourself is that, broadly speaking, the popular understanding of what the research has found doesn't match what the scientists themselves actually conclude. Remember the game Chinese whispers, where one person whispers a phrase, then it gets whispered around the group and inevitably ends up being completely different from how it began? Well, breastfeeding research is a little like that. After the story has been told over and over by people who didn't hear what the original story was, it acquires a life of its own, one in which the advantages of breastfeeding are greatly exaggerated.

Why and how? Well, there are a number of reasons.

Not all studies are created equal

For one, much of the early research into the benefits of breastfeeding didn't factor out things such as a mother's IQ, her age and weight – all things that affect the health of a baby. When those studies from the 1960s and 1970s concluded that breastfed babies were healthier, they didn't recognise that those babies were also healthier because their mums were better educated, older and healthier themselves. But by then it was too late – the mantra 'breast is best' was already born and mothers were already being told that 'research shows that breastfed babies are significantly healthier'.

While modern research is getting better at accounting for these confounders, there is still great variation in the quality of breastfeeding studies. Some examine thousands of children, others fewer than 20.[5] Some ask women about feeding habits contemporaneously, others ask them to recall them from decades before. And again and again in reviews and meta-analyses, scientists complain about the variety of definitions used in the research. Some count babies who were given breast milk just once as being breastfed, putting them in the same category as babies who have been exclusively breastfed for months. The big health bodies know that these problems exist,[6] yet none of these issues over quality ever seem to make it into the reporting of the research, in the media or in breastfeeding promotional material. We are simply told 'research has found . . .'

Sasha says:

As a paediatrician, but also as a mum who breastfed exclusively for a little over four months, I find it fascinating how my daughter's infant feeding would have been classified by a study. Indeed, having read the methods sections of over a hundred feeding studies, it amazes me that in some she would have been classified as 'exclusively breastfed', in some as 'partially breastfed', and yet by others – who included only those infants breastfed for a full year as qualifying for 'breastfed' – as 'exclusively formula-fed'! Clearly, this is going to make things a little tricky for the scientists trying to carry out systematic reviews of the data, as a baby who was breastfed for the same amount of time may appear in any of these three groups depending on the study. Certainly, it pays to read the small print.

Association versus causation

Secondly, it's my guess that a lot of the confusion about breastfeeding's benefits comes about because, as readers (and as writers, trying to simplify the research into a bite-sized article), we mix up association and causation. Yes, many studies find breastfeeding and breast milk to be *associated* with healthier babies, which is to say that breastfed babies tend to be healthier. That's very different from saying that the reason these babies are healthier is because of the way they are fed: in other words, the breastfeeding *causes* them to be healthier. It's like saying that most of the children who got As in their maths exam didn't drink cola at lunch time, but many of those who got a C did. Not drinking cola is associated with getting an A, and drinking cola is associated with getting a C, but it's wrong to say that the children's soft drink habits *caused* their academic outcomes. Perhaps, rather, not drinking cola was a symptom, along with those higher grades, of other significant social factors, such having a healthy and conscientious example set by their parents, or eating a nutritious lunch that helped them to concentrate in the exam. Or maybe it's just that the less bright kids hang out next to the Coke machine.

The thing is, the scientists who do the work know the difference between association and causation, but it just doesn't seem to make its way down to the end readers – us. The most comprehensive review of breastfeeding studies to date, the 2007 AHRQ report for the American government, explicitly states that: 'A history of breastfeeding is associated with a reduced risk of many diseases in infants and mothers from developed countries. *Because almost all the data in this review were gathered from observational studies, one should not infer causality based on these findings*'[7] (my italics).

Let's just think about that for a little bit. This is the most comprehensive review of breastfeeding studies ever conducted, for a government that sets health policy for millions of women and their babies. And what it is saying is that, although breastfed babies are generally healthier, we can't assume that it's the breastfeeding that made them that way. This is a major, radical statement, yet this caveat is nowhere to be found in any of the public messaging around 'breast is best'. Why? Well, we can only assume that because of various social, political and economic reasons, it's been deemed by policy makers that women can't be trusted to sift through nuances. Rather than being told the more complex message, that a broad body of evidence shows us that breastfed babies are healthier than formula-fed ones, but we can't be sure that it's *all* down to the breastfeeding, the more simplistic message is drummed into us. In other words, even though mothers are constantly told that they need to be given all the information in order to make an 'informed choice' about feeding (i.e. to choose to breastfeed), we can only be trusted with the information that reinforces that 'breast is best'.

Circular procedures

Another problem is what American academic Jules Law refers to as 'circular procedures' in his feminist analysis 'The politics of breastfeeding: assessing risk, dividing labor'. Virtually every piece of breastfeeding research starts off with the preamble 'the benefits of breastfeeding are well established'. Never mind that much of the original research into breastfeeding was seriously flawed. Never mind that, actually, there is a lot of conflicting evidence about the benefits of breastfeeding. Simply by virtue of repeating the phrase, authors help build irrefutable 'facts on the ground'. And as Jules Law points out, 'All too often, scientific research into the consequences and effects of infant-feeding choices concludes by acknowledging the inconclusiveness of its own results but then recommends breastfeeding on the grounds that its virtues are already well established in any case.'[8]

So where does that leave you as a parent trying to decipher the truth about breastfeeding's benefits? Confused, I expect. Well, in the next part of this chapter we will look at some of breastfeeding's main touted benefits to show you that the evidence is less clear-cut than you have been led to believe.

Because of the sheer amount of research, it is not possible to provide a comprehensive review of all the literature on breastfeeding here. What we will do, however, is highlight what the most respected, frequently cited studies into its main purported benefits say.[9] (Next time you see a midwife or a doctor, bear in mind that they are unlikely to have read very much of the original research material either – it's not their fault, there's simply too much of it. Also remember that when doctors do find time to read journals, they are more likely to read just the introductory abstract that sums up the article and its findings, rather than the full article that includes all the caveats, the limits to the research and warnings about over-interpretation.[10])

There will necessarily be quite a bit of academic-speak, but hey, you're a smart woman … you can handle it. And knowing for yourself that the research is not as unequivocal as we have been led to believe will hopefully go a long way to banishing that guilt.

'Everyone feels inadequate about something to do with their baby'

Very early on I decided not to let myself feel guilty about bottle-feeding and I did it this way: I decided to just try to be happy.

I couldn't breastfeed. I managed maybe two or three times, but K couldn't latch on, the hospital midwives and nurses were too busy to help, and K's blood sugar dropped, so onto the bottle he went. I kept trying though. A lovely La Leche lady suggested we wait and try syringes of milk till he grew a bit. Then I had a tiny baby who was still really hungry and was now fighting and grazing his mouth on a plastic medicine syringe. I hated every moment, I felt like I was torturing him. So I stopped fighting him in the name of being perfect. He got a bottle and it was all okay. I expressed a bit but that didn't last and that was okay too. I just focused on him and did what I could and we were both great.

I love my family but I really quickly got tired of the daily breastfeeding update. For a month, my mother-in-law continually asked about my boobs and whether I had tried to breastfeed again and whether and how much I was expressing. I hated it. In the end I said that I didn't want to talk about it, but I'm pretty sure she just asked my husband instead.

I have a lovely group of friends I made through NCT but I found one thing really tough. We went out to a cafe with the babies and they were all breastfeeding. There I was scrabbling in my pram for bottles and knocking milk everywhere as I tried to prep a feed. Way to feel inadequate. They were all lovely and sympathetic, but I felt insecure and couldn't help wondering: did they feel superior? I tried not to feel bad and to just get on with things. Within six weeks some of them started asking for advice on bottle-feeding. And then the babies grew a bit, developed at different rates, and I learned that everyone feels inadequate about something to do with their baby. Breast versus bottle just gets more attention.

Sam, London, mother to K, 19 months

Respiratory tract infections

One of the most commonly touted benefits of breastfeeding is that it prevents coughs, colds and various types of respiratory infections, and it is true that the great majority find that breastfeeding is associated with fewer respiratory infections, and with fewer and shorter hospitalisations.[11] This makes sense. Breast milk contains bioactive elements, including immune cells and antibodies that fight common infection-causing bacteria[12] – formula does not have these properties. These elements can help boost a child's resistance to coughs, colds and other respiratory illnesses.

However, there are also some studies that you wouldn't have heard about where the results aren't as clear-cut. Some find breast milk helps to protect only girls, not boys. Others differ on whether it protects the upper or the lower respiratory tract, variously finding that it has a positive effect on one but not the other. One well-conducted piece of research found that breastfeeding doesn't affect chest infections or coughs, or pneumonia at all.[13] Another says that exclusive breastfeeding 'significantly' reduces the duration of a respiratory illness – by that it means it lasts five instead of six days – but doesn't affect the overall risk of contracting one.[14] One widely quoted meta-analysis (a study that brings together several existing studies on the same subject to try to provide a more authoritative analysis) found that bottle-fed babies were three times as likely to be hospitalised for severe respiratory illnesses as breastfed babies,[15] but a very large-scale and well-respected study found that babies who were breastfed longer and more exclusively did not have significantly fewer respiratory infections than those who were breastfed for a shorter time or whose mothers also used formula.[16]

It's also worth noting that even in studies that find breastfeeding protects against certain illnesses, the researchers aren't able to distinguish *how many* were avoided because of these bioactive elements, and how many were avoided because of that X factor of breastfeeding mums tending to have better health practices generally. Quantifying breast milk's protective effect is virtually impossible, not least because it wouldn't be ethical to expose a child to the flu in the name of a science experiment. It is made even more difficult by the fact that breast milk varies in composition from mother to mother, and it also changes throughout the day.

Does breast milk have a 'protective effect' against respiratory tract infections? Yes, a large body of evidence suggests it does. But try to remember that a 'protective effect' doesn't mean that it prevents them. Regardless of whether babies are breastfed or bottle-fed, they can pick up illnesses.

Ear infections

Middle-ear infections are related to respiratory infections because they usually begin with an upper respiratory tract infection (in other words, a common cold) before migrating to the ear. They are very common – nearly half of all children have one before their first birthday.[17]

Parenting tomes frequently tell us that breastfeeding helps prevent middle-ear infections, and while it very likely does, there is not actually full scientific consensus on this. While the majority of studies do find it offers protection, there is disagreement about the *level* of protection, and some studies find it offers none at all.[18]

One study, while finding that 51% of breastfed babies and 76% of formula-fed babies had had otitis media (ear infections) by the age of one, also noted that 'although … human milk has immunologic and non-immunologic protective properties, data from our laboratories and elsewhere do not conclusively show whether breast milk is protective or whether components of formula-feeding are conducive to onset and recurrence of otitis media'.[19] So, the higher rates of ear infections in formula-fed babies could be down to, say, the bottle, the feeding position, the formula, which lacks breast milk's anti-infective properties, or, at least in part, the health behaviours of formula versus breastfeeding parents. Theoretically, if babies are fed in a more upright position (as is advised to avoid ear infections), bottles are prepared and given correctly, and parents make sure they keep their and their babies' hands clean while feeding, could the rate of ear infections in formula-fed kids be reduced somewhat? It's very likely. (We'll talk more about these important ways you can help reduce the likelihood of illness in your bottle-fed baby in Part 2.)

It's also worth pointing out that the biggest factor, other than mode of feeding, in determining middle-ear infections is exposure to group day care, with a number of studies finding it can double a child's chance of getting one.[20] Essentially, the more kids and their germs your child is exposed to, the more likely she is to become unwell.[21] Children in group child care are more likely to be formula-fed than breastfed – an important confounder that not all studies have properly accounted for.

The message we can draw from the research into ear and respiratory infections is that breastfed babies as a group have fewer infections, and breast milk has elements that foster the immune system and act against infection. However, there is no consensus on how much protection it provides, and the simple act of bottle-feeding will not, on its own, result in your baby becoming unwell. The lower rates of infection in breastfed babies could stem, at least in part, from the wider health behaviours of their parents. Regardless of whether you breastfeed or bottle-feed, doing things such as keeping your baby away from masses of people, especially during the winter flu months, dressing her appropriately, and making sure she is handled only by people with clean hands will also help to prevent infection.

Gastrointestinal infections

One claim about the benefits of breastfeeding that is robust and backed up by good evidence is that breastfed babies have fewer gastrointestinal infections. There are a number of large-scale, good-quality studies that all point to breastfed babies having fewer incidents of diarrhoea,[22] and to that effect being *caused* by breastfeeding, not simply *associated* with it. What's more, scientists have a pretty good idea of what leads breastfed babies to have healthier guts. Breast milk contains several properties, including secreted antibodies (IgA – immunoglobulin A), oligosaccharides (small carbohydrate molecules) and lactoferrin, which work by, among other things, helping to stop certain bacteria and viruses sticking to the gut wall.

A very large trial in Belarus that compared babies who were breastfed longer and more exclusively with babies who were breastfed for a shorter duration and in combination with formula found that, in the first year of life, exclusive breastfeeding decreased the risk of gastrointestinal tract infections by 40%.[23]

One good study conducted in England in the 1990s found breastfed babies were four times less likely to suffer from diarrhoea than formula-fed babies, with the strongest protective effect seen when babies came from deprived areas,[24] where there is more overcrowding. The researchers didn't find a magic wand for life, though – the effect seemed to wear off two months after breastfeeding stopped. And the study also pointed out that poor sterilisation of bottles could also be responsible for some of the cases of diarrhoea. Other studies have made the same point.[25] When mothers consistently complain of not being given adequate information about how to prepare bottles safely, including sterilisation, this is a real worry. We'll look at this issue in more depth in Chapter 4, and tell you how to safely sterilise and prepare formula in Part 2.

With all that in mind, the fact remains that breastfed babies, on the whole, have healthier digestive tracts than formula-fed babies, and that is because of breast milk's unique bioactive properties.

Sasha says:

While formula will never be the same as breast milk, a recent randomised controlled trial (the best sort) looked at formula supplemented with bifidobacteria.[26] This is a type of bacteria found in abundance in the guts of breast milk-fed infants and that is thought to contribute to the reduced rate of diarrhoea in these babies. It found that the supplemented formula produced a gut bacterial profile similar to that of the breastfed infants. Even more interestingly, the study showed that use of a formula that was low in phosphate and protein (and therefore more similar to breast milk), even without added bifidobacteria, produced similar results. Currently, no formulas in the UK are supplemented with bifidobacteria because, in order to keep the bacteria alive, formula needs to be made up at 50° Celsius, which is lower than the recommended 70° Celsius needed to kill harmful bacteria. It is possible to buy separate probiotics powder for babies which you can add to cooled bottles, but there are no official guidelines on this, and the effects of these separate powders have not been tested extensively. Speak to your doctor if you're considering supplementing with probiotic powder.

Obesity

This is a big one for researchers (no pun intended), perhaps because it relates to two of modern society's favourite commandments for women: 'Thou shalt breastfeed thy child' and 'Thou shalt not be fat'. (Woe betide the overweight bottle-feeder, condemned to a life of sideways stares and judgement.)

After wading through many of the key journal articles on breastfeeding and obesity, here is the headline: some studies find breastfeeding has a protective effect against being overweight later in life, some don't. Often, the more potential confounders are taken into account, the less of an effect is found, if any at all. Studies with thousands of subjects conducted in Brazil, Hong Kong, Kuwait, Belarus and Britain have all found no correlation between the mode of feeding and childhood obesity.[27] However, plenty of other studies and meta-analyses have[28] (although it must be noted that the quality of research in some of these has been questioned).[29]

A 2011 study that reviewed a lot of the available literature summed up the research well with its woeful title: 'Breastfeeding and body composition in children: will there ever be conclusive empirical evidence for a protective effect against overweight?'[30] (The answer was no.) It concluded that: 'With respect to the avoidance of childhood overweight, strategies aimed at eating or activity habits may be more promising than a breastfeeding promotion.'

Finally, a systematic review published in 2013 – by the World Health Organization (WHO) no less – found a 'small reduction, of about 10%' in the number of overweight or obese kids who were breastfed longer, but it also added that it wasn't possible to rule out other factors being responsible for this. And 'the protective effect of breastfeeding may be overestimated by publication bias and residual confounding'.[31]

It is true that more formula-fed babies are overweight than breastfed ones, but this can largely be accounted for by the demographic differences in their families – breastfeeding mothers generally are wealthier, better educated and, we can assume, healthier. However, where the extra weight can't be accounted for by these different demographics, there are several theories about why formula-fed babies may be more prone to being more overweight than their breastfed counterparts.

One is that formula itself alters the production of several hormones, such as insulin, leptin and adiponectin, which regulate energy use and weight gain[32] in infancy and in later life. This might be due to larger energy intakes in formula-fed babies (see below), but could be brought about by the extra protein in formula compared with breast milk.[33]

Another possibility is that it is the *rate* of weight gain that is important for influencing later weight. Rapid weight gain as a baby, as happens more frequently when formula-feeding, has been shown to make being overweight later in life more likely.[34] Several studies have shown that formula-fed babies consume higher volumes of milk than breastfed babies.[35] One possible cause of this is the way formula-fed babies receive the milk – from a bottle. If the milk is flowing from the bottle too quickly, babies can easily take too much. One recent study suggested that even babies fed expressed breast milk from a bottle gained weight more rapidly than the infants fed at the breast, although the effect was marginal.[36]

Still one more possible reason is that formula-fed babies are less able to tell when they are full than their breastfed counterparts, which could lead to them consuming more than they need. Certainly, as anyone who has been to a first birthday party can tell you, at 12 months formula-fed babies are, on average, half a kilogram heavier than their breastfed friends.[37]

Helping formula-fed babies better tell when they're full – a study

An interesting, if small, study in 2012 tested why breastfed babies may be better able to tell when they've had enough than formula-fed babies.

Researchers added free glutamate to standard cow's milk formula and compared babies' consumption of that with their consumption of regular formula. (Glutamate is an amino acid that signals fullness. It is much more highly concentrated in breast milk than in cow's milk.[38])

The results were fascinating. On average, the babies drank 18% less of the supplemented formula than the regular formula: the added glutamate helped to send the signal to their brain when their tummies were full. The researchers concluded that the findings 'call into question the claim that formula-feeding impairs infants' abilities to self-regulate energy intake' and suggested that adding glutamate to formula could help reduce consumption. In other words, improve the milk and you'll reduce the overfeeding. More research in this area would be very helpful.

It is also pretty obvious that there are lots of other things that occur over many years that relate to weight, such as how much you eat, how much you exercise, and how much television you watch. In fact, the biggest indicator of whether a child is at risk of becoming overweight is not whether she is breastfed or bottle-fed, it is her mother – overweight women are more likely to raise overweight babies.[39]

So what does that mean for you? Certainly it means that formula-feeding alone will not make your baby fat. If you and your partner are healthy and are bottle-feeding sensibly and sensitively, chances are that she will be no more likely to be overweight than if you had breastfed her. For practical tips on how to avoid overfeeding when using a bottle, see Part 2.

Diabetes

When it comes to diabetes, the AHRQ report into breastfeeding and its effects prepared for the US government is a good place to start,[40] as it is extensively quoted in subsequent research and thoroughly assessed in the most authoritative existing literature. After looking at a number of meta-analyses and studies into type 1 diabetes, formerly known as juvenile diabetes, the authors found that 'even though there is some evidence that breastfeeding for more than three months is associated with a reduced risk of type 1 diabetes, this evidence must be interpreted with caution' because of basic problems of quality within the original studies.

One theory is that early exposure to cow's milk protein (the basis of most formulas) can set off type 1 diabetes in people who are genetically predisposed to it.[41] Breast milk may also give a degree of protection in a similar way as it does with gastrointestinal infection – through its transfer of protective immune factors, the body is less likely to be exposed to infections, especially viruses, that are suspected of triggering many types of auto-immune diseases, including type 1 diabetes. However, there are also a number of studies that find no link between the disease and early cow's milk or formula exposure, particularly when parents' diabetes status is taken into account.[42] And one even found that breastfed babies were more likely to develop the condition![43]

The AHRQ report had similar issues with the research into type 2 diabetes. This form of diabetes is closely related to body mass and makes up about 90% of diabetes cases in developed countries. It was previously thought of as being an adult disease, but now is increasingly seen in young people as obesity levels rise. While acknowledging that the studies showed breastfeeding to be associated with a lower risk of type 2 diabetes, the report finds that many failed to account for important confounders like the individual's weight, parental diabetes status, parental class and mother's size. As a consequence, it states that: 'This could lead to an overestimate of the association.' The authors also suggest that publication bias (where studies that show some effect are more likely to be published than studies that show no effect) is 'another possible explanation for the consistent associations observed in these studies'. And again, there are also individual studies that, after taking into account potential confounders, show no relationship between bottle-feeding and type 2 diabetes.[44]

As one piece of research (which did find some links between adolescents with diabetes and bottle-feeding) points out: 'The biologic plausibility for a protective effect of breastfeeding against type 2 diabetes in youth lies primarily in the potential for breastfeeding to reduce the risk for childhood obesity.'[45] Given that obesity is a key trigger for type 2 diabetes, and we have already seen that the link between bottle-feeding and being overweight is questionable, we should be wary of research loudly proclaiming a link between formula and diabetes. The frequently substandard quality of the research linking the two is even more reason to be cautious.

It's the same bottom line as with obesity: stay healthy, don't overfeed your baby, be a generally good parent, and I'll eat my hat if your baby is more prone to diabetes because you formula-fed rather than breast-fed her.

Intelligence

Intelligence is a complicated thing. It is moulded by many factors: some nature and some nurture.[46] The nature side – our genes – we can do little about. The nurture side we can. From birth, a baby's home environment, her diet and her personal experiences all affect her cognitive ability, and these are all within our power as parents to at least partially control.

The role of breast milk and breastfeeding in intelligence has been investigated repeatedly. The great majority of studies find that breastfeeding has a positive effect on IQ.[47] However, yet again reviewers complain of the same methodological problems we keep on running up against – different definitions of what constitutes breastfeeding, inconsistent accounting for important confounders such as maternal IQ, social class and intellectual stimulation, plus there is the persistent inability to factor out the type of parenting provided by mothers who choose to breastfeed. The conclusion of the major research review for the US government in 2007 was that 'there is either little or no evidence for an association between breastfeeding and cognitive performance in children'.[48] Most studies were also conducted before long-chain polyunsaturated fatty acids (LCPUFAs) were routinely added to formula.

One piece of research took a novel approach to the question of whether breastfeeding positively affects intelligence, examining over 6,000 sibling pairs to reduce the chances of differences between families changing the result. By comparing children who had been breastfed with their bottle-fed siblings, it found no effect of breastfeeding on intelligence. What mattered most, in the authors' analysis, was maternal intelligence.[56]

The same conclusions were reached by a smaller paper in 1999 that looked at IQ in children at age 4 and then again at 11. It found 'the observed advantage of breastfeeding on IQ is related to genetic and socio-environmental factors rather than to the nutritional benefits of breastfeeding on neurodevelopment'. Again, maternal IQ and parenting skills were the key determinants of children's intelligence.[57]

I mention these studies to show you that there is conflicting evidence on breastfeeding and IQ. However, the overall trend in the literature is that breastfeeding does affect intelligence. In 2013 the WHO conducted a very thorough review of evidence that put the improvement at 2.19 IQ points on average, after the mother's IQ was taken into account.[58]

Long-chain polyunsaturated fatty acids – worth the money?

There is some debate about whether adding LCPUFAs to formula has a positive effect on intelligence. The main LCPUFAs that are now routinely added to formula are DHA (docosahexaenoic acid), which aids brain development, or ARA (arachidonic acid), which aids eye development.[49] Both are found in abundance in breast milk, but not in cow's milk. The DHAs and ARAs that are added to formula are different in structure from those found in breast milk, and are derived from fish oil, algae and fungus.[50]

Some studies have shown that adding these substances to regular formula has a positive effect on brain development and function,[51] others not. A systematic review of 15 studies for the Cochrane Library (one of the most reliable sources of health information) came to the conclusion that routinely supplementing formula with LCPUFAs could *not* be recommended because the majority of studies they looked at did *not* show a beneficial effect.[52] The authors recommended more trials with a higher dose of DHA. It's important to note that they found no evidence that supplementing causes any harm. Since that review, a high-quality randomised controlled trial has found that children who were fed supplemented formula did better at preschool vocabulary and intelligence tests between the ages of 3 and 6 than those fed regular formula, even though it hadn't been shown to have an effect when the kids were younger.[53] Most of the studies reviewed by the Cochrane Library looked at IQ tests in younger children. This latest, small study suggests that the benefits of supplementation might not be seen until later in childhood. We need more research into this.

There is another possibility, suggested by research in New Zealand, that not all babies metabolise LCPUFAs because of variations in their genes, which could help explain why some respond to supplementation and others don't.[54]

The European Food Safety Authority, WHO and US Food and Drug Administration have all allowed LCPUFAs to be added to formulas, though it is not compulsory. Some organic formulas don't add DHA or AHA because of worries over the chemical used to remove them from the source material, a solvent called hexane.[55]

So where does that leave you when you're trying to debate whether to pay the extra 15% or 30% for the formula with added fatty acids? We can't give you a definitive answer – it's your money, and your baby. At the moment, though, there is some evidence that they can help, and no serious evidence that they harm. There is no evidence that supplemented formula improves brain function more than breast milk, and don't believe any advertising that suggests it does.

There is also a very big 'but'.

As the authors of the biggest ever partially randomised trial into human lactation wrote: 'Even though the treatment difference appears causal [i.e. breastfeeding appears to improve IQ], it remains unclear whether the observed cognitive benefits of breastfeeding are due to some constituent of breast milk or are related to the physical and social interactions inherent in breastfeeding.'[59]

In other words, there are three potential reasons behind improved cognitive performance in breastfed children: the milk itself; the closer interaction between mother and child that breastfeeding provides;[60] and those immeasurable differences in the behaviour of mothers who choose to breastfeed.

The good news is that bottle-feeding parents can attempt to replicate all of these.

First of all, if you have read the conflicting evidence about the effect of adding long-chain polyunsaturated fatty acids and decided it is worth it, you can buy a supplemented formula. When your baby is weaned, feed her oily fish such as salmon, tuna or mackerel twice a week as they are good, naturally occurring sources of fatty acids.

Secondly, interact closely with your baby during feeding, giving her lots of cuddles. We'll go into this more in the segment on bonding (page 66) but actively engaging with your baby during feeding times, as breastfeeding mums tend to do more than bottle-feeding mums,[61] appears to have positive effects on her neurodevelopment. Scientists base this belief on heavily cited research on rats, which shows that the stress responses of rat pups who are 'licked and groomed' by their

---

Sasha says:

Whether a difference in IQ of two to three IQ points would have any real or relevant impact on your child's academic achievements or later career, well-being or happiness is quite another question. Just because a difference is 'statistically' significant does not mean that there will be a clinical or real-life significance to the person or their family.

mothers are permanently altered for the better. It gives rise to the suggestion that 'the physical and/or emotional act of breastfeeding might also lead to permanent physiologic changes that accelerate neurocognitive development'.[62]

Ladies, lick and groom your pups! Show them that you love them! And get their dad to lick and groom them too! Another thing that is believed to improve a child's cognitive and overall development is father interaction, so if you have been unable to breastfeed, try to see it as an opportunity for dads to get more involved in the care of your baby. It's not only good for your sleep, it's good for the little one too.[63]

The best thing to do is simply to be an engaged, attentive, responsive parent full stop. You don't have to breastfeed to do this.

One proven way to boost your child's IQ is to talk to her. A lot. From the moment she is born. In *Brain Rules for Babies*, the developmental molecular biologist John Medina urges parents to speak 2,100 words an hour to their children (which may sound impossible but is actually not that hard – and singing counts too). He quotes research that found that, by age 3, children whose parents regularly talked to them 'had IQ scores 1½ times higher than those kids whose parents talked to them the least'.[64]

He also recommends structured play, and when children do well, praising them for putting in effort, rather than for being smart, as ways to produce intelligent children.[65]

Even the lead author of a recent, very thorough study from Harvard – which suggests that there is not only a link between breastfeeding and intelligence but the more you breastfeed, the higher the IQ boost – told me in an interview that women should not read the results of her study and despair.[66]

Dr Mandy Belfort reassuringly says: 'In our study, the strongest predictor of a child's intelligence was the mother's intelligence, regardless of breastfeeding.

'There are many different things that parents can do to promote their child's development. Reading, having the dad be involved … good routines, especially outside the immediate newborn period … as well as avoiding television, especially under the age of 2 or so.'[67]

To summarise, there is a large body of evidence which suggests that breastfeeding promotes intelligence by a few IQ points. However, the factors that might cause this small improvement are complex, and not simply down to the milk. There are lots of things bottle-feeding parents can try to do to boost their baby's intelligence. The bottom line is, feeding your baby formula will not make her dumb.

Bonding

We are frequently told that breastfeeding promotes 'bonding' between mother and child. As *What to Expect When You're Expecting* says: 'Breastfeeding brings you and your baby together, skin to skin, eye to eye, at least six to eight times a day. The emotional gratification, the intimacy, the sharing of love and pleasure … make for a strong mother–child relationship.'[68] The unspoken corollary of that is that bottle-feeding doesn't promote 'bonding', or that if you don't breastfeed you are going to be less close to your baby. You won't love each other as much or have as deep a link as you would if you fed 'as nature intended'.

Here is the short response to that assertion:

Bullshit.

And here is the long one:

The notion that breastfed babies are automatically closer to their mothers than bottle-fed babies is not only insulting to non-breastfeeding mothers, all fathers and adoptive parents, it is not supported by research. This is yet another one of the many assumptions about breastfeeding that has gone unchallenged for too long.

First of all, let's look into what we mean exactly by 'bonding'. Sometimes it's used to describe the emotional connection of a mother to her baby, known as 'the maternal bond', but it can also describe the two-way connection between parents and child.[71] It's often used interchangeably with 'attachment', which is a well-established and well-understood psychological process.

'Bonding' – a new concept

It may be hard to believe but no one really used the term 'bonding' before the early 1970s, when the concept was proposed by two American paediatricians, John Kennell and Marshall Klaus. They published research that supposedly showed that mothers who experienced 16 extra hours of contact with their infants immediately after birth showed better mothering skills, and their infants did better on developmental tests than babies of mothers who didn't have the prolonged contact.[69] They got the idea from observing the animal world – goats, specifically. Female goats reject their young if they are separated from them for even an hour immediately after birth. The good doctors theorised that humans might have a similar 'sensitive period' when they needed to be with their young in order to foster closeness.

The theory became popular as the men toured hospitals in the United States, educating health professionals about their 'discovery'. It was the 1970s, don't forget, and the smell of free love, peace and a return to nature was lingering heavily in the air. The rejection of medical interventions in favour of the basic human desire for touch struck a chord with parents, at a time when 'natural' childbirth, home births and midwife-led births were also becoming more popular.

By the end of the 1980s, however, the theory of a 'sensitive period' had been widely dismissed by the medical community because of the poor quality of research (the original study was based on just 28 mothers – and, duh, it was inspired by goats).[70] The concept of bonding has stuck, though.

Infant attachment

'Attachment', in infancy, refers to the deep feelings of emotional security a child develops as a result of her relationship with at least one caregiver (not necessarily a mother) who is sensitive and responsive to her needs. A core component of secure attachment is that the primary caregiver is a constant and predictable presence in a child's life. A well-attached child feels she has a safe and reliable base from which to go out and explore the world, and forming good attachments is important for future relationships and for an infant to develop into a happy and secure person later in life. Attachments start to form at around six months.

So where does feeding fit into this? Well, the architect of attachment theory, the British psychoanalyst John Bowlby, observed that the method of feeding – breast or bottle – did not affect the quality of a child's attachments.[72] But finding studies into this area is tricky as there has been relatively little follow-up research.

One study published in 2006 looked at more than 150 mothers and their babies in Arizona.[73] It found no evidence that breastfed babies were more securely attached to their mothers at the age of six months. Unsurprisingly, it was the quality of the mother–child relationship, rather than the feeding method, that determined the child's attachment. The authors did find that breastfeeding mothers were more sensitive to their children's needs, but they concluded that it was because the mothers were more sensitive in the first place that they had chosen to breastfeed, rather than the breastfeeding being the cause of increased sensitivity. (Sensitivity in this context is taken as the promptness, consistency and appropriateness of a mother's responses to her baby's signals.)

The maternal bond

If we take bonding to be how a mother relates to and feels about her child, the 'maternal bond', there is a dearth of research into how the mode of feeding affects it. Surprising, really, given how frequently bonding is cited as a benefit of breastfeeding.

One of the few examples of research is a relatively large-scale study conducted in Wisconsin in 2003.[74] Researchers recorded how both bottle-feeding and breastfeeding mothers reacted to their child when the child was four months old, and again when they were 12 months old. At four months, they found the breastfeeding mothers to have a greater bond with their babies than the bottle-feeding mothers. However, by the child's first birthday that difference had disappeared.

They also examined the two-way relationships between mothers and babies at four and 12 months, rating things such as enthusiasm, visual contact and the quality of verbal interaction. At four months there was no difference between the breastfed and bottle-fed groups. By 12 months the breastfeeding mother–baby pairs scored higher, but the bottle-feeding pairs were all within the normal range of parent–baby relationships. The authors concluded that their results were 'encouraging for non-maternal caregivers and mothers who

'I feel I can bond with my baby a lot easier now because I'm not in pain or stressed'

Due to a complicated birth, I wasn't able to attempt to feed April for almost 24 hours after she was born. When I eventually did try she just wouldn't latch on to my breast. Even with the help of several midwives, my poor little screaming baby just would not latch. Feeding times became a cycle of me attempting to latch her, her screaming, me calling the midwives, the midwives attempting to latch her, her screaming, eventually giving up and feeding her expressed milk, then expressing some milk for next time. This process would take around an hour. Sometimes, after much struggling, she would latch on and then lazily feed for an hour or so, meaning the process took even longer.

She was on a strict three-hourly feeding schedule (due to her having lost so much weight), so by the time I got her settled after a feed and expressed some milk, it was almost time to start over again. I had a few complications during and after the labour, which meant I was in a lot of pain and had to take good care of myself. I was really struggling to see how I could take care of my baby and look after myself at the same time. I was exhausted.

After being in the hospital for a week, we were discharged and I promised the midwives I would continue to try to breastfeed her. But once I got home, I was just so exhausted I decided I would express milk and feed her with a bottle instead. She would still be getting all the benefits of breast milk, just from a bottle. It was a bit of a hassle expressing many times a day, but compared with trying to breastfeed her it was easy.

After five weeks of successfully feeding her expressed milk, I got a bout of mastitis. It was very painful and I felt absolutely rotten. Antibiotics cleared it up in a few days; however, it came back a week later with a vengeance. The ducts became so blocked that my supply in my left

continued

continued from previous page

breast dropped to almost nothing. I had to start supplementing with formula. It took me a couple of weeks, several ultrasound therapies and another course of antibiotics to clear the ducts this time around. But just when I thought I was in the clear, it came back again. This time, I was over it. I decided the pain, the doctor and physio visits, the antibiotics and not to mention the time spent expressing and trying to massage out the blockage were just not worth it. I switched to formula full time and I do not regret it one bit. My baby is happy and healthy and so am I. I feel I can bond with her a lot easier now because I am not upset, in pain, or stressed. To me, bonding with my baby is also an important part of keeping her healthy.

Cara, Perth, Australia, mother to April, 4 months

bottle-feed their children … [It] reminds us that maternal care is a complex set of behaviors and attitudes robust enough to persist and remain adequate despite *minor deviations* from its original or natural form'[75] (my italics).

Finally, a 2008 systematic review of all the scientific literature looking at breastfeeding, infant attachment and maternal bonding found that 'assumptions of a positive role of breastfeeding on the mother–infant relationship are not supported by empirical evidence'.[76]

The authors of this very thorough review added that they are not ruling out that there may be some effect, but more and better research should be done into the area. They point out that, theoretically, what could encourage caring behaviours and therefore bonding in mothers are the breastfeeding hormones oxytocin and prolactin.

The role of oxytocin in bonding

Oxytocin, as you'll remember from your antenatal class, is known as the 'love hormone' and its release has been shown to promote trust[77] and reduce maternal stress.[78] It circulates during vaginal birth and breastfeeding, but also during skin-to-skin contact with your baby. If you're worried that you're potentially missing out on some loving feelings by not breastfeeding, make sure you have lots of cuddles with your little one, and, even better, make it skin to skin.

Neuroscientist and child psychologist Bruce Perry, the founder of the Child Trauma Academy in the US, has these other suggestions:

> ❝The acts of holding, rocking, singing, feeding, gazing, kissing and other nurturing behaviours involved in caring for infants and young children are bonding experiences. Factors crucial to bonding include time together (in childhood, quantity does matter!), face-to-face interactions, eye contact, physical proximity, touch and other primary sensory experiences such as smell, sound, and taste. Scientists believe the most important factor in creating attachment is positive physical contact (e.g. hugging, holding, and rocking). It should be no surprise that holding, gazing, smiling, kissing, singing, and laughing all cause specific neurochemical activities in the brain. These neurochemical activities lead to normal organization of brain systems that are responsible for attachment.[79]❞

As Bruce Perry mentions, feeding is a great opportunity to bond with your baby. (Notice he doesn't say breastfeeding or bottle-feeding? That's because it doesn't matter!) Really try to 'tune in' to your baby during a bottle-feed, as this 'sensitivity' is believed to be one of the aspects of breastfeeding that promotes positive parenting and closeness.[80] It's easy to give a bottle while Facebooking, talking on the phone or reading a magazine (trust me, I know). But for at least some of the feed, try to really focus on your baby. Hold her close, be very attentive to her hunger signals (don't just shove the bottle in and keep it in) and try to get some good eye contact.

The bottom line of all this is don't get your knickers in a twist about bonding. Ultimately, you know yourself whether breastfeeding makes you feel closer to your baby, and your baby feel closer to you. For a mother who enjoys breastfeeding, it can be an uplifting, even ecstatic, feeling that enhances her connection. However, if you're someone who doesn't enjoy it, do not be fooled into thinking that just keeping your baby at your boob is going to create a closer relationship. It might, but what is just as likely is that you'll end up being grumpy and resentful every time a feed rolls around.

> ## Sasha says:
> And for those women who are unable to directly breastfeed their infants for any number of reasons, it is also important to remember this message: there are few things sadder than a new mum who is so focused on her child getting breast milk that she is stuck to a breast pump all day and thus unable to cuddle, play with and 'bond' with her child as she would want to. We each need to weigh the benefits of breast milk against the costs, and if one of those costs is spending more time with your pump than your child, I would encourage you to remember that what babies need more than anything is a loving and present mother.

The maternal bond and infant attachment all develop over time, and through many facets of your daily interaction. Research and plain old common sense show you that you are not condemning yourself to an inferior relationship with your child if you don't breastfeed. You will find other ways to create the bond between the two of you, by playing, singing, cuddling or through a myriad of other activities. Personally, I found just staring into my daughter's eyes as I gave her a bottle to be an incredibly emotionally bonding experience, as did my husband when he fed her. And when she reached up with her little hand to touch my face as she was sucking away, there was really no feeling like it.

A few myths busted

Breastfeeding gets mothers back in shape faster

We've all heard about those famed 500 calories a day that breastfeeding supposedly burns – it's one of the biggest carrots held out to new mums. Many a celebrity credits their incredible post-baby bodies to breastfeeding. Well, the real story is, it's only partially true (and there is even conflicting evidence on that). The AHRQ systematic review of studies into the area found that 'the overall effect of breastfeeding on return-to-pre-pregnancy weight (1 to 2 years postpartum) was negligible'.[81] One of the studies they looked at did find breastfeeding women achieved their pre-pregnancy weights about six months earlier than bottle-feeders, but overall they found that household income, pre-baby weight, ethnicity and energy intake were all bigger factors. It makes sense – while it's true that breastfeeding does burn up calories, what those baby books don't tell you is that it also can make you incredibly hungry! That was a point made by one researcher who published a small study that found that non-lactating mothers actually lost *more* weight at six months than their lactating sisters. She wondered if the breastfeeding hormone prolactin, which stimulates appetite, caused breastfeeding mums to overeat. Or maybe it was because non-breastfeeders were more able to exercise[82] (which was certainly true in my case). Either way, the jury is out. If you want to lose your baby weight, the best advice is probably just to lay off the doughnuts.

Giving your baby any formula means they will never exclusively breastfeed

New mothers are often warned that giving their babies a bottle of formula early on will decrease their chances of successful breastfeeding because breastfeeding relies on supply and demand to get established, and babies exposed to bottles might come to prefer them because they get the milk faster and more easily. It can be very worrying for women dealing with a hungry, crying baby who is losing weight because their milk hasn't 'come in' but they really want to breastfeed. A small, but high-quality, study published in 2013 found the opposite – that early, limited formula use may actually increase your chances of being able to breastfeed for longer overall.[83] This randomised controlled study tested the use of small amounts of formula milk to 'top up' after breastfeeding in the first week until a mother's breast milk production became established. The results showed that doing this significantly increased the number of babies being exclusively breastfed at three months. The top-ups were done via a syringe, not a bottle, and were limited to 10 ml per feed – a very small amount fed in a very specific way. Given that research has found that nearly half of all American first-time mothers wait longer than three days for their milk to come in,[84] and that concern over lack of milk is the biggest reason for women giving up breastfeeding, it's time that we busted this myth that giving *any* formula to tide over a hungry baby until mum is producing enough will ruin breastfeeding forever.

Breast milk is 'pure', formula is 'poison'

Breast milk is sterile, whereas formula (except for ready-to-feed bottles) is not. Breast milk is also packed with lots of nutrients, antibodies and all sorts of good stuff, the majority of which aren't found in formula. But that doesn't mean it's 'pure'. Breast milk picks up environmental contaminants, so in a modern world, that means it also contains paint thinners, dry-cleaning fluids, wood preservatives, toilet deodorisers, rocket fuel, termite poisons and flame retardants.[85] The amounts are microscopic and, in the overwhelming majority, not harmful, and, according to Florence Williams' excellent book *Breasts*, 'Some studies have found that breast-fed babies develop better despite the additional chemicals found in breast milk, which is why the World Health Organization . . . recommend[s] breastfeeding even among the Inuit, whose breast milk could technically qualify as hazardous waste.'[86] But is something that technically qualifies as hazardous waste 'pure'? I don't think so. As for the idea that formula is poison, anyone who makes such an absurd statement should immediately be ignored. They are clearly fools. Formula is one of the most highly regulated foods in the world. It provides protein, energy, fats, vitamins and minerals and has turned out generations of perfectly healthy human beings. Nuff said.

Formula-feeding is expensive but breastfeeding is free

Let's get one thing straight: breastfeeding is not free, people! It is physically and emotionally demanding, and if you need some help to get it right, it can in fact be bloody expensive (see 'Breastfeeding – an emerging big business' on page 88). Aside from the costs of lactation consultants, breast pads and breast pumps, if you're lucky enough to have breastfeeding fall into place with a minimum of fuss it still has financial implications. A 2012 American study found that women who breastfed for six months or longer suffered more severe and longer earnings losses than mothers who breastfed for a shorter time or women who used formula.[87] Part of the reason for this, the researchers posited, is because breastfeeding isn't protected enough at work, and maternity provisions in the US are bad. Both are certainly true, and the damage to future earnings of breastfeeding women could potentially be offset if the right to breastfeed (and I do see it as a right) were better defended. But that doesn't change the fact that breastfeeding is only 'free' if a woman's time and energy are worth nothing.

Dr Mandy Belfort, a Harvard researcher whose 2013 paper found a correlation between breastfeeding and intelligence (so hardly a cheerleader for formula), took me by surprise when she said to me in an interview: 'I think the costs of breastfeeding have never been truly measured correctly, and it's very hard to weigh up costs and benefits when you don't have a measure of costs. The financial costs of equipment, pumps, workplaces creating private places for women to express their milk . . . the need to maybe get some extra help around the house, help with other children, the reduced productivity at work – those are all costs that you can put a dollar value on. And we just need to say how much it costs, in addition to how much value we're getting, how much health we're buying.'[88] I couldn't have put it better myself.

A final word on scientific research

Good science is vital to understanding and improving our world. Substandard science clouds our understanding and can even be harmful. In this chapter we've looked at how frequently research into breastfeeding and formula-feeding isn't up to scratch, and also how research findings have been misinterpreted in public health messages. We have only had the space to go into a few of the purported benefits of breastfeeding, but hopefully what we have presented has shown you that when you see a poster proclaiming 'breast is best', you're getting a very simplistic message that has a much more complicated backstory.

Researchers point out that breast milk is very complex and we are only just beginning to understand it. That is true. In time, with large-scale, well-designed studies, researchers may well be able to prove the extent of the benefits of breastfeeding. But we're not there yet, and overzealous breastfeeding advocates should stop saying we are.

You won't be surprised to find out that problems of poor study design and over-interpretation are not limited only to breastfeeding research. There is growing concern that research in all fields is getting less robust, as scientists compete for funding and career enhancement, journals lower standards for publication and researchers struggle to keep up with the latest statistical modelling.[89] There have been major flaws found in the peer-review system, which is supposed to rigorously check studies to make sure they are up to scratch before being published.[90] The scientific community is aware that there is a problem, and some organisations are trying to do something about it.[91] But remember too that science is not conducted in a vacuum. As long as tests are devised and performed by humans, with all our prejudices and fallibilities, there will always be some imperfections. How much do those imperfections matter? In the case of breastfeeding research, where babies' health and mothers' well-being are at stake, they matter a lot.

Breast milk *is* better than formula. We know that. The question is, is it so much better that the pressure currently put on women to breastfeed no matter what the cost to their mental and physical health can be justified? Based on the evidence we have reviewed in this chapter, we would argue it's not. Encouragement and support of breastfeeding? Yes. Recognition of the modest benefits of breastfeeding in developed countries? Yes. A one-size-fits-all approach that pressures women to breastfeed no matter what their personal circumstances? No.

When I was visiting my parents in my small, rural home town recently I paid a visit to my old paediatrician. He had looked after me, my two sisters and most of the local kids in his 43-year career as a children's specialist. Hilary Mercer is his name. Despite being nearly 70 and recovering from lymphoma, he's still practising. He's one of those doctors who just loves his job.

I wanted to get his view on the differences between formula-fed and breastfed children, bearing in mind that because we live in a small town he has known his patients not only as babies, but as children, teenagers and now adults with kids of their own.

So I asked him, over coffee and biscuits, could he tell the difference between a breastfed child and a formula-fed one?

He looked me squarely in the eye. 'Nope,' he replied. 'Can you?'

'Well, I can't,' I said, 'but I'm not a doctor or a nurse. I can just go by the kids in the playground.'

He elaborated: 'Look, on a clinical level in trials, it's possible to see some differences, but don't forget those researchers are *looking* for differences. On a practical level . . . I can't tell.'

It echoes a comment I read on www.parenting.com from Dr Nancy Butte, Professor of Paediatrics at Baylor College of Medicine in Texas, who has been studying breast milk and formula for 20 years. 'It's hard to distinguish between a well-cared-for bottle-fed infant and one who's breastfed,' she told the website.[92]

And that seems to be the factor that we're missing as we endlessly debate what study found what, and whether the evidence is reliable – it's the *care* of the baby that matters most. As the bottle-feeding support group Bottle Babies says on its website, 'How you fill their tummy is not as important as how you fill their heart, mind and spirit.'[93]

3 The Breast-feeding Echo Chamber

How everything you read reinforces 'breast is best'

Every once in a while I have difficult conversations. They go a lot like this one, which I had with a male fellow journalist friend, when we caught up for a drink recently.

Joe[1]: So what are you up to now?

Me: Well, I'm actually writing a book about why women shouldn't feel guilty if they don't breastfeed.

Joe: Right . . .

Me: It's not anti-breastfeeding. It's just pointing out that some of its benefits have been overstated and we need to get a bit more balance into breastfeeding promotion.

Joe: But it *is* better, Mad. There's all that research. And I just read the other week about how breastfeeding can even prevent autism. And Alzheimer's. And my wife loved breastfeeding.

Me: I'm sure she did. I liked it too. That's awesome – breastfeeding's great when it works. But have you read these studies? Because I have, and I can tell you they're a lot more nuanced than what the NHS and the newspapers say.

Joe: No, I haven't read them myself, but ... Are you saying the WHO is wrong?

Me: No, but the WHO recommends health policy for developing countries too, where the benefits of breastfeeding are that much more important than here. You can see why it promotes it so heavily. And actually, yes. Some of the claims the WHO makes on some of its websites and documents *do* overstate the benefits.

Joe: <falls off chair>

These conversations are hard for me. I am no conspiracy theorist. I passionately believe in science, vaccinations, public health, and the work of the WHO and UNICEF. I have spent a lot of time working in developing countries where their work is crucial. But, in some people's minds, pointing out that maybe breastfeeding isn't quite what it's cracked up to be puts me on the same side as climate-change deniers and the nutbags who think that AIDS is just a big corporate conspiracy.

But Joe's response is entirely reasonable. After all, why would anyone think that breast milk is anything other than liquid gold? It's the message we get every time we go to the GP, open the paper or look on a parenting website. Joe, like pretty much all of us, has been caught up in the Breastfeeding Echo Chamber, where breastfeeding's benefits have been magnified and repeated so loudly and so many times that the only message we can hear through all the noise is 'breast is best'.

In this chapter we'll break down the cultural and media contexts in which this message is spread. Our aim is to give you some critical thinking tools, so the next time you read a blog or an article about breastfeeding's unquestionable superiority, you'll be more able to judge its accuracy for yourself.

To do this, we'll first look at how the modern lactivist movement was born out of the shameful history of formula companies. In the process, you'll see that despite what some breastfeeding advocates say, there has always been a need and a desire for mothers to find ways to feed their babies other than via their own breasts.

We'll then look at how sloppy reporting of breastfeeding science by mainstream media contributes to an outsized impression of its benefits, and why that latest story about how breastfeeding stops you from getting acne or Asperger's may not be entirely accurate.

Next, we'll look at the role the internet is playing in shaping our views not only about feeding but about motherhood. We'll examine three of its biggest pitfalls – the proliferation of inaccurate information, how parenting extremists are setting new parameters for what is 'normal', and the creation of online parenting tribes at war with one another.

Finally, we'll take a look at how celebrities are shaping our views about feeding our babies, and why looking to them for inspiration is not always the wisest choice.

A quick history of breastfeeding and the alternatives

While some breastfeeding extremists would have us believe that outsourcing baby-feeding only began with big profit-hungry corporations, women have needed alternatives to breastfeeding since time began. In fact, advice for treating lactation failure is mentioned in the earliest medical encyclopaedia, written in Egypt in 1550 BC.[2] Forget about fenugreek and massaging your breasts in the shower, if women were low in supply in ancient Egypt, they were told to rub the bones of a swordfish on their backs, or eat 'fragrant bread of soused durra', while rubbing their breasts with a poppy plant. (Whether these ladies suddenly burst forth with ounces of breast milk isn't recorded. If you would like to do your own experiment, please go ahead and let me know the results!)

When the swordfish bones weren't doing the trick, a wet nurse was the first port of call. If not the oldest profession, it's definitely the second oldest, and wet nurses have been literally saving lives for millennia.

But bottles and substitute milks have always been used too – feeding vessels made out of clay with a nipple-shaped spout were found in babies' graves as far back as 2000 BC.[3] Until the invention of a hygienic bottle in the Industrial Revolution, though, this was a dangerous proposition. Our ancestors didn't understand that germs spread disease, and even as late as the early nineteenth century, it's estimated that one-third of all babies who weren't breastfed died.[4]

There are no accurate figures for how many women couldn't or wouldn't breastfeed throughout the ages, but historians have uncovered a few pieces of information. For example, it's believed that around 20% of the wives of American plantation owners during the slavery era used a wet nurse to either fully or partially breastfeed their babies.[5] There has always been a need, and in some cases a desire, for a woman to find another way to feed her baby other than at her own breast.

But women who don't breastfeed for whatever reason have also always been criticised. In post-revolutionary America, they were considered to be selfish and unpatriotic.[6] In the Middle Ages, people worried that wet nurses could pass on illness through their breast milk, illness that the baby could then pass on to the parents.[7] Getting canned for not breastfeeding is nothing new, it's just that the reasons for it have changed.

Introducing formula

The seeds for the widespread use of formula we see today were first planted when the first patented infant formula was invented in 1865.[8] Others soon followed, but formula and bottles really took off at the start of the twentieth century, when paediatricians decided that advising women on feeding babies was a good way of boosting their income, and, therefore, something they needed to be much more involved in. Even though these (nearly always male) doctors advised that breastfeeding was best, they still recommended formula as a good

'I mixed-fed from a bottle because my daughter never managed to latch on'

I was planning on breastfeeding my daughter, but Maisie was never able to latch on. In hospital, a number of breastfeeding specialists all agreed that my technique was perfect and that there was plenty of milk available. But as Maisie didn't seem to be able to get anything out, they showed me how to manually extract the colostrum and put it in a syringe and squirt it in her mouth. However, I knew this wasn't keeping her full.

Once at home, I again demonstrated my breastfeeding technique to the health visitors. It was always described as faultless, and I was just told to keep on trying and given the numbers of various helplines (which I never had time to ring). But as it was quite clear that Maisie never managed to ingest any milk, to keep her alive I immediately had to make the decision to bottle-feed her. I really wanted her to have breast milk, primarily to boost her immune system, so from the first day I returned home I spent four or five hours a day on the breast pump, managing to express as much as 70% of her daily feed, the rest being formula. I was only able to do this because I had my mum around during the day once my husband had returned to work. I was determined to keep this up for as long as possible, but after a couple of months (and several broken breast pumps!) my mum was no longer available, and with no other daytime support I had to give up expressing. From then on I fed my daughter formula exclusively. I don't have fond memories of that time, and the hours spent on the breast pump certainly didn't help.

I felt there were many positives about bottle- or formula-feeding – it meant that I could schedule the feeds regularly, and that both my husband and my mum could feed Maisie, which was something they were keen to do, and I believe that it helped to build the incredibly strong bonds that they still have with her. I think we're incredibly fortunate that we have the option of a safe alternative to breast milk in the West. It terrifies me to think what might have happened to my daughter if formula hadn't been available for the first six months of her life.

Sophie, London, mother to Maisie, 2 years

option, and particularly liked it because it meant they could regulate and supervise feeds, medicalising what had, until then, been women's business. Meanwhile, formula companies advised that their products should be used only with a doctor's prescription, creating a symbiotic relationship.[9] However, just as today, some women were also grateful for the liberation from their bodies that bottle-feeding provided.[10]

Two world wars saw many more women start to work outside the home, and at the same time science and technology began providing ever more popular solutions to the labour-intensive 'women's work' of the past. Modernity was all the rage, and, gradually, we reached a point in the 1950s when only about half of all new mothers in Britain were even attempting to breastfeed,[11] and only a quarter of American mothers.[12] Breastfeeding looked as though it was on its way out in the rich world. But a group of Catholic housewives in Chicago wasn't going to let it go down without a fight.

Breastfeeders fight back

In 1956, seven Chicagoan women came together to form La Leche League and set about promoting their core belief that: 'Mothering through breastfeeding is the most natural and effective way of understanding and satisfying the needs of the baby.'[13] (The name La Leche League came from a statue in Florida honouring Nuestra Señora de la Leche y Buen Parto – or Our Lady of Happy Delivery and Plentiful Milk. LLL used the codename because, at the time, even using the word 'breastfeeding' was a no-no. It is now the largest breastfeeding organisation in the world, active in over 70 countries. It has consultative status with UNICEF and is regularly consulted by the WHO on breastfeeding matters.[14])

These housewives are generally credited with being the pioneering force in bringing back breastfeeding from the threat of extinction. In the late 1960s and early 1970s, their movement coincided with the hippy movement and a pushback against medicalised childbirth and child rearing. Their promotion of breastfeeding was rooted in ideology rather than science, but it was at this time that studies started coming out showing that breastfed children were healthier[15] than their bottle-fed counterparts. But these studies often didn't account for the factors such as a mother's IQ, health, age, wealth, etc. that we have seen make the differences appear bigger between bottle-fed and breastfed babies.

The formula companies then signed their own death warrant in the court of public opinion when they were outed for their unconscionable marketing practices in poor countries in the 1970s. Companies, including Nestlé, had been hiring women to dress up as 'Mothercraft' nurses and give away free formula samples to new mothers. When the mothers' breast milk dried up, they were left reliant on expensive formula. In developing countries, clean water and the sterile conditions that are needed to safely prepare formula are frequently not found. Add to that the fact that women were soon watering down the formula to make it go further, and babies began suffering. Babies became malnourished and some died. It was a scandal, and although Nestlé eventually won a libel action against a charity that called formula 'the baby killer', the damage was done, both to breastfeeding in the developing world and to the image of formula. From then on, formula companies would be forever struggling to rid themselves of the notion that they take advantage of women and harm babies.

This abhorrent marketing in poor countries helped start a worldwide movement to protect and encourage breastfeeding, and in 1981 the World Health Assembly adopted the International Code of Marketing of Breast-milk Substitutes. The voluntary code restricts formula marketing – it's the reason for the 'breast is best' warnings on formula tins, and why you'll never see (in a signatory country) advertising for formula for children under the age of six months. It's also why in Britain, Australia and New Zealand you'll never be given free samples of formula, though in the United States, which isn't a signatory, parents can be.

Since then, the international community, led by UNICEF and the WHO, has taken more steps to shore up support for breastfeeding. The global goal of exclusive breastfeeding for four to six months (later amended to six) was decided at a big UNICEF/WHO meeting in 1990, at which the Innocenti Declaration on the Protection, Promotion and Support of Breastfeeding was signed. The document declared that 'attainment of this goal requires, in many countries, the reinforcement of a "breastfeeding culture" and its vigorous defence against incursions of a "bottle-feeding culture"'.[23] The battle to promote breastfeeding had begun in earnest, and there was no question about who were the goodies and the baddies: on one side, UNICEF and the WHO standing up for exploited women and unprotected babies; on the other,

Breast and formula-feeding in developed and developing countries – what's the difference?

The global push for breastfeeding has been driven largely by UNICEF and the WHO, and gathered steam after the formula scandals in the developing world in the 1970s. All the international codes, declarations and initiatives on promoting breastfeeding nearly always give the same policies for rich and poor countries, even though there are some very major differences in the importance and impact of breastfeeding versus formula-feeding in the different settings.

Despite great improvements in recent decades, many people living in poor countries still don't have access to clean water or good sanitation,[16] which are crucial for making up bottles safely. Diarrhoea is one of the leading causes of death for children under 5 worldwide,[17] and UNICEF estimates that a formula-fed child living in diseased and unhygienic conditions is at least six times more likely to die from diarrhoea than a breastfed child.[18] Formula is also comparatively much more expensive, so mothers are more likely to water down powder, leading to malnutrition. Clearly, in these settings, promoting and supporting breastfeeding are crucial not only to the health but potentially to the life or death of a child.

Because of the relative importance of breastfeeding in settings of poverty, there are different recommendations for breastfeeding women with HIV in rich and poor countries. In the developing world, the risks of formula-feeding without clean water, sterilised equipment and guaranteed formula supply are considered more dangerous to a baby's health than the possible transition of the virus through a mother's breast milk, so breastfeeding, with HIV drugs, is recommended.[19] In rich countries, where formula-feeding is much safer, the risk of HIV transmission through breast milk is considered the greater danger, so HIV-positive women are recommended to formula-feed.[20]

Immoral marketing from formula companies is not the only reason why women don't breastfeed in developing countries – there are widespread cultural beliefs that impact on the uptake and duration of breastfeeding as well. For example, in India, there is a common belief that colostrum is harmful for babies so it is usually thrown away,[21] even though breastfeeding itself is very common. In Liberia, which has one of the world's lowest breastfeeding rates, there are widespread myths, such as that breastfeeding while pregnant weakens the foetus, that a woman shouldn't breastfeed if a previous child died while it was being breastfed, and even that women can't have sex while breastfeeding because semen mixes into the breast milk, making it dangerous for the child. Because women want to be able to satisfy their husbands and not risk being abandoned, they choose to give up breastfeeding instead, and give rice and water, which is their traditional alternative to breast milk.[22]

Breastfeeding is also not necessarily always easier in a poor country than in a rich one. Poor people still get inverted nipples, insufficient glandular tissue and postnatal depression. If they don't have support networks to help, or breastfeeding role models, they might struggle in the same way as a British or Australian woman could without help. Those famous 500 calories a day that breastfeeding burns up might be the only calories a woman in a poor country gets, meaning she has to choose between nourishing herself and nourishing a child. And a woman who can barely feed herself is definitely not going to be able to afford formula, safe bottles and sterilising equipment. Although UN agencies rightly proclaim that hundreds of thousands of babies in the developing world die because of suboptimal breastfeeding, in many cases that suboptimal breastfeeding is a symptom of the poverty and lack of agency that rules a woman's entire life, rather than simply an outcome of pushy marketing.

multinational corporations responsible for creating a 'bottle-feeding culture', and that were only worried about their bottom line.

Formula's understandable image problem

Sadly, many formula companies are still living up to the image of the bad guys by continuing to engage in predatory marketing in poor countries. In Indonesia, they give gifts to midwives, along with samples of formula, and the media have reported that midwives even have sales targets for formula, in clear contravention of the UN code on marketing.[24]

In Turkey, a 2013 investigation by the UK's Bureau of Investigative Journalism found formula company Danone (which makes Milupa, Aptamil and Turkish brand Bebelac) was conducting a campaign erroneously telling women that their babies needed 500 ml of breast milk a day after the age of six months, and if mothers were worried that babies weren't getting enough, they should top up with formula.[25] Despite the fact that no public health body recommends a minimum amount that babies should be consuming, the campaign was a commercial success. The 'outreach', according to the company's annual report, 'addressed a major public health issue and simultaneously energised the Turkish infant formula market, generating 15% growth in formulas designed for children aged 6 to 18 months'.[26] Danone insists it follows the WHO recommendation of promoting exclusive breastfeeding for the first six months and says it has contributed to a 17-year rise in rates of exclusive breastfeeding. However, giving out incorrect information about nutritional needs for babies in a manner designed to boost sales is at least unethical, if not strictly in contravention of the code on marketing.

A third example: a 2007 film by UNICEF showed how widespread television marketing and the use of gifts to health workers in the Philippines had convinced mothers that expensive formula was better for their babies than breast milk. It told of how doctors and nurses were given gifts and incentives for recommending certain formulas, and how women were sent home from hospital with free formula samples, which is against the law. The film recorded mothers of young babies watching advertisements for formula that glamorised the product. One featured a child musical prodigy playing to a packed audience – the clear message being that formula will make your baby smarter. Despite the widespread lack of clean water and the huge comparative cost of formula, Filipina mothers were convinced they were doing better by their children by not breastfeeding.[27]

These are just a few examples – there are many more. I was personally shocked when a Chinese friend told me during a recent trip to Beijing that she was still giving her 18-month-old four bottles of formula a day because 'he needed it', and that she had moved from breastfeeding to formula because it was better. This from a fiercely intelligent, sharp journalist, in a country that has been beset by formula scandals – it shows the power of marketing. It's no wonder that industry analysts are predicting that the Chinese formula market will double in the next three years.[28]

Buying from these companies

It's impossible not to feel furious at formula companies for continuing to put profit before babies' health and even lives, and not only because of the damage it does to mothers and children in the developing world. When the big brands continue to act like assholes, where does that put us, formula-feeding mums, in the public view other than in league with the corporate baddies? How can we trust companies that deliberately try to undermine breastfeeding? Quite simply, we can't, and that has huge negative follow-on effects in terms of the perception of formula as a substance, the perception of formula-feeders, and public policy around information on formula.

Suzanne Barston, one of the pioneering voices 'standing up for formula-feeders without being a boob about it', as her blog's subtitle proclaims,[29] illustrates the bind eloquently in her excellent book *Bottled Up: How the Way We Feed Babies Has Come to Define Motherhood, and Why It Shouldn't*:

> 66*[Formula companies'] actions have caused a reverse halo effect, making it difficult for some to separate the product from the producer. Formula as a substance did not convince women that their bodies weren't capable of nurturing life; marketing executives, injustices and bad circumstances did a bang-up job of that all on their own. Formula as a substance does not kill babies; the water used to reconstitute it does – rather than blame the powder sitting in the can, we should be blaming the infrastructure.*99

By infrastructure, she means the lack of clean water, sanitation, maternal education and the sheer poverty that make formula-feeding a dangerous choice for much of the world.

However, until formula companies clean up their act, despite the fact that they can't be blamed for the poverty that can make formula feeding more risky in poor countries, they will continue to be justly criticised for their poor behaviour. And sadly, formula-feeding parents will continue to be tainted by association. Unfortuntately, with the global market for formula worth $9 billion[30] in 2010 (or $30 billion if you prefer the UN figure),[31] companies will continue to seek out the grey (and not so grey) areas of international policies on breastfeeding marketing to promote their product.

So if we accept, as we do and should, that breastfeeding should be promoted and protected, then we do need safeguards, which is what international organisations and policies aim to provide. Despite 50 years of concerted breastfeeding promotion, around the world only two in five babies are exclusively breastfed for six months, and that figure has been stable for a couple of decades.[32] However, even though formula companies are still pushing their products in morally questionable ways, we should remember that there are many complex reasons why women can't or choose not to follow the international guidelines, and they are not always simply because they have been won over by an advertising campaign.

And while we do definitely need those safeguards against predatory formula promotion, their unfortunate side effect has been the damaging conspiracy of silence around how to safely use formula in countries such as Britain, Australia and New Zealand, and the general demonisation of formula and formula-feeding mothers.

Breastfeeding – an emerging big business

Public promotion of breastfeeding, originally started to counteract the power of the big formula companies, has spawned its own cottage industries in recent decades. While minuscule in scale compared with the estimated $9 billion formula market,[33] the lactation consultant, nursing aids and pumping industries are nonetheless growing in size in response to the needs of women who want their babies to have breast milk but are having trouble.

There are over 26,500 International Board Certified Lactation Consultants (IBCLCs) in 96 countries.[34] The IBCLC qualification is the gold standard for this still relatively new profession. (The certifying body was set up in 1985.) IBCLCs are free to charge what they like for the skills and knowledge they bring in helping women to breastfeed, and sometimes the cost can run to more than £150 for one consultation.[35] Many women swear by them, but others have paid for numerous lactation consultants with no luck. There are also many breastfeeding counsellors who operate on a voluntary basis.

It may seem hard to believe given its ubiquity, but pumping is a relatively recent phenomenon too. Medela, the market leader for breast pumps and other breasty paraphernalia was established in 1961, and in 50 years it has ballooned into a hugely profitable, multinational corporation. When its top-of-the-range breast pump retails for £200 plus, it's not hard to see why.

Then there are the nipple shields (£8), nursing pads (£10) and nursing bras (£29 for two from M&S) as well as the books on breastfeeding (running at 3,000+ on Amazon last time I checked).

Unless you need to see a lactation consultant several times, the total cost will never be as much as feeding your baby formula for the first six months of her life, but breastfeeding can certainly end up being a costly exercise for something that is supposed to be free and come naturally.

Sloppy science reporting

Now that you have a better understanding of how the global campaign to promote breastfeeding came about, let's look at what role the media plays in keeping the 'breast is best' message bouncing around the Breastfeeding Echo Chamber.

I have a Google alert for 'breastfeeding'. Every day, I get sent at least one article telling me about a new study finding a new benefit, making reason 1,542 why women should do it, just in case you hadn't got the message already. It makes me want to tear my hair out, not because I am against research into breastfeeding and formula, or reporting on that research, or against breastfeeding – it's just that so much of the reporting of these studies is so crappy.

As you have seen from Chapter 2, research into breastfeeding is a complicated thing, with many caveats and pitfalls. Thankfully, scientists are getting a lot better at trying to account for the many factors that could skew research findings. Journalists, sadly, don't seem to be getting much better at reporting the nuances, though. Thanks to my research into breastfeeding literature, I know better than to believe every single headline, but why would parents of a new baby who have just made the sometimes difficult decision to start using formula do anything other than believe every word of what they read? And when you're in a sleep-deprived, emotional state, each of these stories can feel like just one more nail in the guilt coffin.

Well, here is some news that you are unlikely to see in the papers: the Breastfeeding Echo Chamber is fuelled by an epidemic of sloppy science reporting that unquestioningly reproduces press releases from universities and journals without bothering to check the limitations of that research, the credentials of the researchers, or sometimes even what the research has actually found. I know, because I'm sorry to say that in my 15-year career as a journalist I have done my fair share of sloppy science reporting (though thankfully not on breastfeeding).

As Joan B. Wolf found in *Is Breast Best?* after taking an in-depth look at how the media report on science:

66Research also demonstrates that medical journalists are more likely to allow certain subjects, such as doctors or scientists, to state hypotheses unopposed; that they rarely question methodology, a starting point for evaluating research; and that they tend to rely on syndicated news packages and media information produced by health centres, drug companies, and other vested-interest groups. One study found that press releases from prominent medical journals circulated to reporters 'frequently presented data in exaggerated formats, and failed to highlight study limitations or conflicts of interest'.[36] 99

This comes as no surprise to me. As someone who works in the media, I am, sadly, all too aware of journalists' shortcomings, and how press officers looking to get research into the public domain are able to exploit them – and, if needs be, amp up what their research has actually found in order to get coverage.

How research gets picked up by the media

Here's how it works. You're a reporter under pressure to file for tomorrow's paper or for the next news bulletin and you've got nothing. Suddenly, you're saved by an incoming press release for a story about a fantastic breakthrough – a scientific journal is publishing a story that breastfeeding has been found to prevent (insert terrible affliction here). Hooray! You read the one-page press release. If you are assiduous and you have time, you read the abstract (the brief description of the study and its findings), then you call up the researcher (who is keen to plug their work and their amazing finding) for a 10-minute interview. Do you read the study itself where it talks about the limitations of the research? No way – no time for that, and you can't properly interpret statistics anyway. Do you write a headline that says 'A small sample suggests a possible link between breastfeeding and x, but more research is needed'. Hell no! Who would read that?! You write 'Link found between breastfeeding and prevention of x' or, if you are a little more sensationalist, you write 'Breastfeeding prevents x'. You file and, job done, you can go home. And your editor is happy because everyone loves a story about medical breakthroughs, especially ones that confirm what we already know – that 'breast is best'.

Of course, there are some great science and health reporters out there who do know their stuff and do a far more assiduous and nuanced job, but due to cutbacks in newsrooms across the world, more and more health reporting is falling to generalists who don't know how to read science literature or don't have time to.

Sasha says:

Errors of interpretation occur at every level of reporting. As the much-respected author of *Bad Science*, Ben Goldacre, pointed out when writing in the *Guardian* in 2009, academic press releases are often highly flawed. He points to a study from Dartmouth Medical School in New Hampshire that examined press releases from the most highly respected institutions over one year. One-quarter did not state how many participants the study included and a third did not give numerical figures for their results. Fewer than one in five were high-quality studies using a randomised controlled trial methodology or were a meta-analysis. Clearly, we cannot just lay the blame at the feet of medical journalists if the information coming to them out of the academic centres is limited, incomplete and even misrepresentative.

One person who has made it her mission to cast a critical eye over parenting news is Polly Palumbo, PhD. She runs the Momma Data blog. As a psychologist and former researcher, as well as a mum, she has the tools that us regular old news consumers lack to look behind the headlines and analyse research. And her assessment isn't great.

'Typically, the problem with the more mainstream news organisations involves a lack of nuance rather than outright false information,' she told me.

> **❝**Every day I come across articles even in the more respected news organisations that might, for a number of reasons and in a number of ways, miscommunicate or misrepresent scientific research. There's often a lack of context. It starts with the dramatic headlines and continues through to the exaggerated conclusions. The study gets stretched in significance, its results or importance overstated in subtle ways. On less newsy sites, including many popular parenting sites, accuracy becomes even more problematic, with false information all too common.**❞**

I hear you, Polly.

How research is sensationalised

Let me give you a detailed example of how sloppy science reporting creates a false impression about research. Bear with me, this is going to take a while.

In 2013 a small study in the *Journal of Alzheimer's Disease* looked at a possible link between breastfeeding and a reduced risk of the mother developing Alzheimer's later in life. The study was based on interviews with 81 women aged between 70 and 100, half of whom had dementia. It asked them to recall whether they breastfed, how long they breastfed for, and then matched that up with data about their dementia, along with other factors like their educational and socio-economic status. It found that breastfeeding did have a 'significant' protective effect on developing Alzheimer's for women with no family history of the disease; it had no significant protective effect if there was dementia already in the family. Specifically, it found that a woman who breastfed for a total of 12 months reduced her chance of developing Alzheimer's by one-fifth when compared with a woman who breastfed for 4½ months. On the simple comparison of women who didn't breastfeed at all versus those who did (regardless of the duration or family history), researchers found the women who did breastfeed had a 64% reduction in their Alzheimer's degree risk.[37] The scientists theorised that it could be due to the effect breastfeeding has on oestrogen and/or insulin sensitivity.

Looking at those findings, it certainly seems like a big deal, and, as the researchers note, the potential links are definitely worthy of further study. The newspapers thought it was a big deal too, with most major dailies in the UK carrying the story. But there are a couple of reasons why we shouldn't all be breaking out the nursing bras just yet. For one, the investigators spoke to only 81 women – a small number for any sort of health research. Secondly, the scientists asked the women to recall feeding practices from 40 to 60 years ago, and HALF OF THEM HAD DEMENTIA! (The researchers also did interviews with family and friends to try to corroborate what the ladies told them about breastfeeding practices, but that is still second-hand recall of events from 50 years ago.)

More generally, terms used in science literature don't have the same meaning as how we might interpret them when used in everyday language. For example, if a finding is 'statistically significant', that doesn't necessarily mean it will have what we might consider to be a significant impact in real life. When scientists say that breastfeeding is 'protective against' something, or has 'a protective effect', that doesn't necessarily mean that it will prevent said disease from occurring, simply that the risk is reduced. And we've already talked about the difference between association and causation, and how often we mix them up.

Bearing all that in mind, would you make a definitive statement about breastfeeding preventing Alzheimer's based on this one study? No, and neither would the researchers. That didn't stop the *Daily Mail* though: 'Mothers who breastfed slash their risk of developing Alzheimer's by TWO-THIRDS, claims study,'[38] the paper screamed. Oh brother. This is a classic example of taking one statistic from a very small study and extrapolating it out into a blanket health statement. At no point did the study claim that breastfeeding cut mothers' risk of developing Alzheimer's by two-thirds. No researcher worth their salt would make such a sweeping, definitive statement on the basis of such a small study, and, in fact, the head of research at Alzheimer's Research UK expressed exactly the same sentiments in the article. 'Preliminary studies like this one are important for highlighting associations worthy of further study, but we shouldn't be quick to jump to conclusions quite yet,' said Dr Simon Ridley. But you'd only know that if you read the very last paragraph in the story, because that's where his quote was.

At least the *Daily Mail* went to the trouble of speaking to someone not connected with the study to give a bit of perspective, unlike a number of news organisations that appeared to simply paraphrase the press release.[39] These included Britain's *Telegraph*, whose headline was 'Breastfeeding "lowers Alzheimer's risk"', and the *Huffington Post* with its story 'Breastfeeding may slash Alzheimer's risk, study finds'.[40] Both reports also failed to mention that the results were based on interviews with elderly women, half of whom were not all there. In other reports about the research there were similar faults, but none as glaring as the headline from NaturalNews.com: 'Breastfeeding proven to lower risk of Alzheimer's in moms.'[41] Um ... no it hasn't.

The 'Behind the Headlines' service of the NHS was so concerned about reporting of this study that it ran an analysis piece to try to correct misconceptions. Its conclusion: 'Overall, this study provides some limited evidence of an association between breastfeeding, length of time spent breastfeeding and the risk of Alzheimer's disease. It does not provide evidence of a direct cause and effect relationship, only that there seems to be an association.' Therefore, 'headlines such as "Breastfeeding 'lowers Alzheimer's risk'" ... do not accurately reflect the findings of this study.'[42]

It's a brave attempt to correct misreporting, but the phrase 'shutting the gate after the horse has bolted' springs to mind.

Something else to bear in mind when reading reports about studies like this is the absolute risk of the problem occurring. If you go back and read all the reports in the British media about this study, you'll notice that not once do we learn how common dementia is, probably because it wasn't on the press release. (Okay, that was bitchy – but probably true.) The only figure given is that 'breastfeeding women slashed their risk of Alzheimer's by two-thirds'.

This is an issue that also really irks Polly Palumbo.

> 66The media often report results in relative risks or terms: for example, 'kids not breastfed are 200% more likely to have ear infections' or 'breastfeeding cuts risk of ear infections in half'. These terms don't help parents figure out how this applies to their own lives. It doesn't tell them specifically how many fewer ear infections they can expect if they breastfeed . . . Without this information, what statisticians call absolute risks, it's difficult to put the results into perspective. Is the difference between 1.5 and 3 ear infections [as a theoretical example] meaningful or important to parents? I suppose it depends on the particular parent or child.99

In contrast, when confronted with the equivalent relative risk of 200%, most would naturally think that would be very significant. It's not exactly scaremongering, but it's not giving a true picture that parents can relate to.

To go back to the Alzheimer's study, for the record, according to the Alzheimer's Society, in Britain these are the numbers of people with the disease: 40–64-year-olds – 1 in 1,400; 65–69-year-olds – 1 in 100; 70–79-year-olds – 1 in 25; and 80-year-olds and over – 1 in 6.[43] Whether you consider those figures of serious enough concern to warrant potentially changing your breastfeeding behaviours is entirely up to you. The point is, without being given those absolute risks, we can't make an informed decision.

Does the media ever manage *balanced* reporting?

The prevailing discourse of assumptions about what is good (breastfeeding) and what is bad (bottle-feeding) can even be seen on the very rare occasions when a report suggests that maybe formula is *not* the source of all evil. I had to laugh when I saw a headline from Reuters, which was syndicated in multiple news outlets, entitled 'Formula-fed babies don't always overeat: study'.[44] In reporting what is essentially a good piece of news (how a small study found that by adding an amino acid to formula, babies appeared to be able to tell better when they were full), the headline sets it up with a false claim – that formula-fed babies *always* overeat. Not only does the piece of research being discussed not make that statement, no piece of research ever in the whole wide world has found that formula-fed babies *always* overeat. But the headline, which has no factual basis, reinforces a misconception.

The other frustrating habit of the news media can be seen in reporting on studies that are published showing *no* positive relationship between breastfeeding and a particular outcome. Here, the tendency is to list all other benefits of breastfeeding, just in case mums read one story and decide on that basis that there's no reason to keep up with this nursing lark. For example, in covering research that showed *no* association between breastfeeding and obesity, an Associated Press article opened by drawing attention to breastfeeding's 'many benefits'. It featured a quote from the study's lead author saying, 'I'm the first to say breastfeeding is good,' even if it has no impact on obesity.[45] This is the same 'circular procedure' US academic Jules Law described when talking about scientific research into breastfeeding.

The tendency to always remind us of breastfeeding's benefits is complemented by the media's habit of reminding us of formula's 'risks'. In a feature detailing one mum's struggle with breastfeeding and her terrible treatment by NHS midwives entitled 'When breast is not necessarily best: huge pressure put on today's mothers to breastfeed their babies. One woman's haunting tale reveals how it can lead to great anguish', a newspaper managed to turn a rare critique of breastfeeding promotion into a dig at formula. At the bottom of the piece in which a mother comes to the conclusion that, in her case, formula was best, the *Daily Mail* added this helpful info box:

> **"**AND TO COMPOUND HER WORRIES: THIS IS WHAT GOES INTO FORMULA MILK. To create a product doctors, scientists and manufacturers agree is vastly inferior to breast milk, powdered formula needs 46 ingredients including preservatives, emulsifiers, stabilisers and supplements. But it still lacks ingredients that help promote brain growth and antibodies.[46]**"**

It then goes on to list all those terrible ingredients and how crap they are compared with breast milk. The box has no relevance whatsoever to the story, other than to say: 'Well, this poor love may well have had a terrible time, but let's not forget that formula is poison.'

Formula-feeding mums: if it feels like just about the whole media is against you, I'm afraid that's because it generally is. Breastfeeding advocates rightly say that women still face huge barriers to breastfeeding, but the news media is not one of them. It's not as though there is some big conspiracy to make us feel bad, it's just that there is a combination of powerful habits: reporting on breastfeeding studies without fully understanding or adequately representing the research, and always driving home the message that 'breast is best', even if the main thrust of the story is neutral or negative about breastfeeding.

That said, in the past few years there has been a growing number of comment pieces defending a woman's right to formula-feed. However, most of them focus on the aspect of choice, rather than pointing out that maybe we're not getting the full, nuanced picture about the benefits of breastfeeding from either our media or even our doctors. And why would any journalist bother to put their heads above the parapet and question the status quo? Those who do, such as Hanna Rosin, who wrote the seminal 'Case against breastfeeding' for *The Atlantic*,[47] just get slammed for it – in Rosin's case, five years on. (NOTE TO SELF: why am I writing this book again?)

It would be good if the media could start to look a little deeper into the latest piece of breastfeeding research before reporting it, but I'm not holding my breath. So, in the meantime, friends, next time you read about the latest amazing discovery about why breast milk is so superior and how you are raising a second-class human if you subject your baby to formula, take a deep breath. The story and the research itself could both be top class, factual and correct. We do know, after all, that breast milk *is* better than formula and breastfed babies do tend to be healthier. But history shows that the media have a less than stellar history in reporting the nuances of scientific research in general, and breastfeeding research in particular.[48] So before you jump off a bridge, email the researcher, look up the study yourself – it may well be online – look for other media reports. You might just be hearing some loud reverberations from the Breastfeeding Echo Chamber.

The pitfalls of the internet

Of course, these days we don't get information just from newspapers and TV. The vast majority of women in rich countries use the internet to make decisions about pregnancy and childrearing.[49]

The internet is a wonderful place. It has given us unfettered access to information, given the voiceless and marginalised a platform, and has created parenting communities across continents. But, as always in life, there are flip sides. And these flip sides – the pitfalls of the internet – all contribute to the Breastfeeding Echo Chamber and the negative image of bottle-feeding.

Pitfall 1: More information doesn't mean good information

When anyone with a modem can set themselves up as an 'expert', misinformation becomes scarily commonplace, and this is particularly true when it comes to information about bottle-feeding. There are plenty of websites out there (which I won't name because I don't want to up their hit rate or cause you to make a hole in the wall with your head) that are filled with ABSOLUTE BOLLOCKS about formula and its 'dangers'. Don't let a professional appearance fool you. If you find a website informing you about how formula will destroy a baby's 'virgin gut',[50] or one telling you how 'no one can make you feel guilty without your consent', or one that refers to Defensive Formula-feeders, STEP AWAY FROM THE COMPUTER, LADY. Those are all the classic warning signs that you are going to get nothing but trouble from that particular URL.

There are three main sources of information about bottle-feeding on the internet: formula companies, breastfeeding sites and official health bodies. This is a problem. Formula companies are clearly not coming from an objective point of view, and while they will tell you about the wonders of their product, there is no comparison with other companies' formulas to help you make an informed decision. Information on formula preparation and how to feed tends to be basic and doesn't emphasise the important emotional and physical aspects of feeding. And can we really trust their guides about how much babies need when it is in their interests to sell more product? I'm sceptical.

Then we get to the breastfeeding sites, which have two subgroups: 1) sites that tell you why you *shouldn't* be using formula; and 2) more neutral sites (including the big baby sites such as babycentre.com) that, while emphasising that 'breast is best' (just in case we'd forgotten), give information of varying quality about formula and how to use it. Given that a study of breastfeeding sites in 2006 found that only seven out of 30 met all the quality criteria set by the American Academy of Pediatrics in relation to information about breastfeeding,[51] what standards do you expect about information relating to something that they are trying to discourage? Breastfeeding sites invariably overplay the health benefits of breastfeeding and regularly talk about the 'risks' of formula. Plus, given how quickly poorly reported studies about breastfeeding and bottle-feeding in particular, and health more generally, filter through the internet and quickly become 'fact', that leaves us facing an avalanche of misleading advice that can seem overwhelming.

Official health sites, such as the NHS Choices[52] site or the Australian government's 'Pregnancy, Birth and Baby',[53] do have useful information, but for curious parents who want more than just a simple 'how to' guide, they are light in content, and they are often not what appears first in a Google search.

Dr Karleen Gribble, an Australian-based breastfeeding advocate and researcher who is an active participant in internet discussions on feeding issues, agrees. As she told me over email:

> **❝**The quality of information on infant feeding is a real mixed bag. On breastfeeding there is probably more information in total and a decent amount that is good quality. On formula-feeding, things are really patchy. There's lots of really awful

*info – much is from industry sources and even the stuff that is
really good and practical doesn't provide the level of detail
that I think is needed. In my opinion, parents don't need to just
know the how of formula-feeding but the why of each step.* **"**

Help is emerging . . .

In the last couple of years, bloggers and ordinary mums have stepped up
to try to fill in the gaping holes. The two leaders are Bottle Babies, started
by Australian mum Lisa Watson, and Fearless Formula Feeder, which is
the internet identity of Californian blogger and author of *Bottled Up: How
the Way We Feed Babies Has Come to Define Motherhood, and Why It
Shouldn't* Suzanne Barston.

Lisa Watson had just given birth to her second bottle-fed baby in 2009
when she set up 'a little Facebook page to try to connect parents to one
another. I saw a real need for bottle-feeding families to connect with
other bottle-feeding families so they knew they weren't alone. Because
I felt alone,' she told me from her home in Queensland.[54] She also saw a
massive information gap.

'There's a lot of support for breastfeeding mums, which is fantastic
because they need it, but when it comes to support for bottle-feeding
parents it's very difficult to find. So much of the information is so spread
out, and it's also very contradictory and surrounded by 'breast is best'
information, which is fine, people need to make an informed decision.
But once that decision has been made, being told all the time that
one way is better than another when you're just trying to find practical
information can be very difficult.'

Bottle Babies is now the world's first charity dedicated to supporting
bottle-feeding families and offers peer support and information sharing
on its Facebook page, administered by volunteers.

Suzanne Barston started her Fearless Formula Feeder blog the same year,
in response to the same lack of information, but also to work through her
own guilt about not being able to breastfeed. Suzanne also helps facilitate
peer support, but her main focus is advocacy around bottle-feeding
issues. This has won her a lot of fans, but also a lot of detractors. 'I've
been called stupid, the c-word, the b-word,' she says matter-of-factly. 'But
for every piece of hate mail, I get 10 emails from people who have been
helped by hearing the stories of other women who are on the blog too.'[55]

'The things I get the most hits on are very practical things like how long
can I keep a bottle out, differences between formulas, what are the best
baby bottles, and drying up breast milk. And I'm not a doctor, I research
a lot, but I'm a writer, so it still really angers me that if you Google those
things I'm still one of the first things that come up. That's a problem.'[56]

Despite the growing acknowledgement of the lack of reliable information for bottle-feeding parents, there is still a huge information gap. We are trying to help correct that with some practical advice in Part 2, and in the Resources section of this book we list a number of good sites for bottle-feeding advice and information.

> ## Sasha says:
>
> As a paediatrician I've met a lot of parents who have been misinformed, or are simply confused by conflicting information from the internet. It can be hard even with medical experience to unpick the useful and robust sites from the poor quality, biased or frankly damaging blogs and websites that exist. It is one of our aims to set out clear and helpful information about bottle-feeding here in this book, and to list other useful and trustworthy resources where further information can be found.

Pitfall 2: The extremists shout the loudest

'I'm a fairly middle-of-the-road parent who's happy to go with the flow, and I'm already really busy and exhausted looking after the kids, but I think I'll invest time and resources to set up my own parenting blog,' *said no one ever.*

By definition, people who have bothered to set up their own blog, website or Facebook group feel pretty passionately about something. With over 4 million mummy blogs, that is a lot of noise about kids and parenting. And what an even cursory perusal of these sites makes obvious is that a fair share of that noise is coming from people who practise parenting styles that may have previously been seen as unorthodox or extreme, because people who were marginalised in their own geographical communities now have a place where they can safely talk about their beliefs.

The rise of attachment parenting is a case in point. Attachment parenting, as pioneered by American paediatrician Dr William Sears, essentially believes that for a child to develop properly it needs to be in close proximity to a parent (usually a mother) in the early years. In practice, it typically means the three Bs: bed sharing, where the child sleeps in the parents' bed for as long as she wants; extending breastfeeding, usually past the age of 2; and baby wearing, where parents keep the infant as close as possible, often in a sling. It is a very child-centred approach to looking after kids. The first time many people heard about attachment parenting was after *Time* magazine's cover 'Are you mom enough', which featured attachment parent Jamie-Lynne Grumet breastfeeding her 3-year-old son while he stood on a stool. However, attachment parenting has been around since Dr Sears published his AP bible *The Baby Book* in 1992, and, many would argue, long before that.

While attachment parenting might not always necessarily be described as extreme (intense would perhaps be a better word), some of its practitioners are. American actress Mayim Bialik, of *Big Bang Theory* fame, breastfed her 2-year-old every two hours through the night, because that's what he wanted. She also didn't allow her 5-year-old to watch TV and had no outside childcare[57] for her kids, despite both her and her husband working. She practised 'elimination communication', where babies don't wear nappies but rather parents try to pick up on a baby's signals of needing to wee or poo. Bialik denies that any of these are extreme, but it sounds pretty full-on to me.

In the internet age, Mayim Bialik and other outspoken AP practitioners enjoy a large platform from which to share their views, in the form of blogs, Facebook and Twitter, forums and websites. Attachment parents are big users of technology, according to Dr Charlotte Faircloth of the University of Kent's Centre for Parenting Culture Studies, who studied attachment parents for her book *Militant Lactivism?* They are typically older, wealthier and very well educated, giving them time and resources to discuss, defend and promote their choices online. At the time of writing, a Google search for 'attachment parenting' yielded nearly 8,500,000 results, many of them news stories, but also many Facebook groups, blogs and organisational sites. Attachment parents take up an outsized portion of the internet, relative to their actual number. If we follow Suzanne Barston's analogy of the internet as the modern equivalent of the town square, attachment parents have set up a large, well-resourced stall at Speakers' Corner, with plenty of high-profile advocates to make their case. This is changing our ideas about what is 'normal', including in relation to how we feed our babies.

But what we forget as we idly cruise the internet is that the people who run the parenting blogs, who set up and moderate the Facebook groups, are not 'normal' – they are passionate by definition. Breastfeeding websites such as KellyMom, in response to the question 'Is weaning going too fast for baby?', reply with quotes from Dr William Sears, the attachment parenting guru: 'certain behaviours of children; i.e. aloofness, aggression, excessive whininess … may all be "diseases" of premature weaning.'[58] So if I stop breastfeeding 'prematurely' (i.e. before her second birthday in Sears' eyes), my kid is going to be a pain in the arse? Righto then … It may just make us roll our eyes, but when a mainstream breastfeeding website is quoting attachment parenting books, that has a trickle-down effect on the women searching for answers. Online life is different from real life, but as we increasingly go online to search for parenting ideas, the more extreme norms that we find online are being transplanted back into our everyday realities.

I'm not trying to pick on attachment parenting here – helicopter parenting, 'tiger mums' and 'unschooling', to name just a few, are all being given a wider audience by the internet. The more we hear about them, the less unusual they become. And what they all have in common is that they place many more demands on parents. And that is fine – every mother and father are completely entitled to parent their child in whatever way fits their values and works for them. But because they're shouting so loudly, we can't help but hear and be influenced by their views. The well-documented shift towards 'intensive mothering', 'total motherhood' or 'the new momism'[59] as described by a number of sociologists, feminists and thinkers (and as discussed further in Chapter 4) is real, and the internet is facilitating that shift ever more quickly. The effect is that our idea about what is normal or acceptable is shifting too. I'm knackered just thinking about it.

Sasha says:

Some of these 'extreme' blogs are really terrifying because they are not written by lunatics or idiots. They are written by reasonably intelligent, sometimes very eloquent, and well-researched individuals. But what they don't do is give a balanced view. These bloggers use their sites to clamour for their individual opinion, and often use valid scientific data to back up those views. The problem is, they're usually only presenting one side of the scientific story, and completely ignoring other research that doesn't fit in with their opinion. I would advise you to avoid reading these blogs. They exist simply to force their views on others and usually, in the case of the breast/bottle-feeding debate, serve up a huge helping of guilt for anyone who feels or acts differently to them. They are so unhelpful for tired, stressed women looking for advice in one of the most difficult periods of their lives.

Pitfall 3: Tribes at war

This pitfall is related to the one above. Increasingly, the internet is where we go to socialise, chat and learn new ideas. As our physical communities and extended families break down, they are being replaced by online communities and families. But rather than these communities being defined by bloodlines or by which street we live on, they are set by our choices and our beliefs. In relation to feeding babies, that has upsides and downsides.

The upside is that we can get support, advice and friendships online that we can't get anywhere else. Lisa Watson, the founder of Bottle Babies, didn't know anyone else who used formula in her mothers' group or even in her town. When she set up the Bottle Babies Facebook page she created the community that she had been missing, and that greatly improved her life.[60] For me, being part of the Bottle Babies community, as well as other Facebook support groups for bottle-feeding parents, has been a lifeline. It's given me practical information, emotional support, and somewhere not to feel judged. And those are all really important.

But the flip side is the silo effect of internet communities – that because we have found our tribe, or tribes, we stick together, reinforcing our beliefs, our prejudices and our practices so that we become less and less able to see the value in different approaches and points of view.

As Charlotte Faircloth of the Centre for Parenting Culture Studies at the University of Kent says:

> **❝**One of the sad things about this tribalisation is that your average mum and dad just can't get along. I think because parenting has become so moralised, it's like, well, are you a formula-feeder or a breastfeeder? Do you use a pushchair or a sling? It's these small and fairly insignificant choices about how

we raise our children that have come to stand for something much, much bigger. About what kind of orientation you have towards the world.[61] **"**

Suzanne Barston recognises that she has become a de facto tribal leader via her Fearless Formula Feeder blog, but it's not something she is comfortable with.

"*It's something I take very seriously and try to take responsibility for. But a lot of other tribal leaders . . . have really encouraged bullying, us against them . . . And one thing I don't like is when people are like, 'I'm a fearless formula-feeder,' because what I really don't want is people identifying themselves by how they're feeding their child.*[62] **"**

There are people trying to bridge the tribal divides. Breastfeeding advocate and attachment parent Jamie-Lynne Grumet (yes, she of the *Time* magazine cover fame) wrote a fantastic blog post entitled '10 things breastfeeding advocates need to stop saying' to formula-feeding parents. My favourite: 'I just think formula-feeding moms are lazy,' to which Jamie-Lynne counters, 'And I just think you're an asshole.'[63] Along with Suzanne Barston and blogger Kim Simons, Jamie-Lynne set up the #ISupportYou movement to try to get breastfeeding and bottle-feeding parents to show support for one another. It was a success, with hundreds of women posting photos of themselves breastfeeding or bottle-feeding with messages of support for the other side.[64]

But that's a rare call for peace in the bottle/breast tribal war. And the fact is that with breastfeeding communities being far more represented online than bottle-feeding communities, it's a pretty one-sided battle. And man, there are some nasty, judgey pieces of work out there.

We all need support networks and communities, and for mums who find they're the only one in the park whipping out a bottle, online communities are invaluable. The same could equally be said of the only woman in the park whipping out her breast. We need to be careful though, not to fall into the 'us versus them' and 'breast versus bottle' trap. In the grand scheme of things, how we feed our babies matters so little, and it should certainly not identify who we are as mothers or human beings. The best advice we can give is: find your people, get support from your people, but don't think that just because you do things one way, that's the best way for everyone. Don't be the troll, and definitely don't feed the troll – they only bite back. Don't bother wasting time on sites or with groups where you'll just get negative comments for your feeding choice. There are much better things you can do with your time, like being with your baby. The faster we can recognise that all parents need support, regardless of how they feed their babies, the better off we'll all be.

'I felt like a second-class citizen because I was no longer breastfeeding'

Within a few days of giving birth to my boy, he was feeding like a champion, even though I had had a breast reduction 17 years ago. But after two bouts of mastitis and surgery to remove an abscess, my breastfeeding journey came to an abrupt halt when my boy was nine weeks old.

Luckily, he took to the bottle immediately, and I made it clear to all my family that I would be the primary feeder, as I felt that if I was breastfeeding it would be my job 95% of the time. I loved feeding my boy and spending that beautiful time with him.

I learned a lot when I began my formula journey, not least about the nasty little world of breast versus bottle. I got absolutely no help from health workers when I had to start using bottles, just a 'continue feeding him' attitude. I felt like I was suddenly a second-class citizen because I was no longer breastfeeding. Luckily, my mum is a midwife and paediatric nurse and my sister formula-fed both her boys, so they helped with my millions of questions regarding bottles, formula, processes, etc.

continued

CASE STUDY

continued from previous page

Anyone who says formula-feeding is easy doesn't know what they are talking about. Formula-feeding is HARD work – there are bottles to sterilise, formula to spoon into bottles, kettles to boil, the list goes on. Plus packing a nappy bag requires a few million items instead of just nappies or clothes. Breastfeeding, while difficult at first, once you get the hang of it and if you have good supply – it's easy!

To mums who are struggling with guilt over using formula, I would say being a mum is so much more than whether we breastfeed or formula-feed. It's about loving our babies and enjoying every moment with them. My boy is now 7½ months old and very happy. In five years' time, no one will be able to tell the formula-fed babies from the breastfed babies, so hold your head high and be proud. You're a wonderful mum, so just love your baby!

Skye, Western Australia, mother to Joshua, 7½ months

Attack of the celebrity breastfeeders

Poor Kate Middleton. As if she didn't have enough to contend with dealing with the pregnancy hormones, a husband who works away, the entire world watching to see if she's developed cankles and the small matter of incubating the heir to the British monarchy, she also had to deal with breastfeeding advocates talking about her 'royal orbs' in the newspaper and how important it was that she set an example and breastfed.[65] And we ordinary folk think we have to deal with feeding pressure!

According to *Telegraph* columnist Beverley Turner's piece in June 2013, the lack of high-profile breastfeeding mothers was contributing to breastfeeding being out of fashion (and therefore why she implored the Duchess of Cambridge to 'get her Royal orbs out').'

What a load of rubbish! Celebrity breastfeeding is the latest addition to the Breastfeeding Echo Chamber as celebrities influence and refine our ideas about what constitutes a 'perfect' mother. They are so ubiquitous you can't have a shameless peek at a celebrity website these days without reading about the latest new Hollywood mum, gushing over the special bond she's getting from breastfeeding her baby. The irony is that in the same Google alert that featured the 'Royal orbs' story, I got links to three different articles talking about how much Kim Kardashian 'loves breastfeeding',[66] is a 'lean, mean breastfeeding machine'[67] and is breastfeeding baby North 'like crazy!'[68]

In their book, *The Mommy Myth: The Idealization of Motherhood and How It Has Undermined All Women*, Susan J. Douglas and Meredith W. Michaels devote an entire chapter to the 'Attack of the celebrity moms'.[69] It charts the rise of the celebrity mother magazine profile from the 1980s (I know – unbelievably, celebrities didn't really talk much about motherhood before then) to the 2000s. They observe: 'Profiles of celebrities ... equated motherhood with winning the Nobel Prize, climbing Mount Everest and experiencing a transforming religious experience, all at once ... No ambivalence, not even a mouse-squeak of it, was permitted. Celebrity moms loved their kids unconditionally all the time; they loved being mothers all the time.'[70]

Douglas and Michaels wrote their book back in 2004 and things have changed since then. It's no longer enough for a celebrity mum to succeed in her career and have a wonderful partner and perfect kids whom she absolutely adores and who have changed her life. That's become far too de rigueur. These days she needs to be all of these things while being 'natural and perfect',[71] and that means, of course, breastfeeding.

Idealised images

There are the celebrity breastfeeding 'selfie' fans – stand up model Miranda Kerr and singer Pink. The breastfeeding magazine cover girls – Angelina Jolie, that's you. The ill-thought-out commentators – Gisele Bündchen and her famous quip that there should be a 'world-wide law' that all new mothers should breastfeed for six months.

Then there are the extended breastfeeding evangelists – Mayim Bialik, Alanis Morissette and Alicia Silverstone, to name a few. And the celebrity mums who are pretty low key about breastfeeding – Maggie Gyllenhaal, Gwen Stefani, Selma Blair. As far as I can tell, the internet went into meltdown when Beyoncé was *reported* to have breastfed her daughter Blue Ivy in a New York restaurant.

And all of this is genuinely great. We absolutely need more celebrities talking about breastfeeding, and especially putting their money where their babies' mouths are and breastfeeding in public. In Britain in particular we could do with more celebrities doing more with their 15 minutes and helping to normalise breastfeeding by doing it in the open. (We could do with more women doing that full stop, which is why, when I was breastfeeding, I made a point of doing it in front of friends, family, at cafes and in parks. Even though my pitifully small amount of breast milk wasn't doing much to sustain my baby, I thought I could at least strike a blow for normalising nursing in public.)

But if breastfeeding advocates think that hearing another famous person gushing about nursing is going to improve breastfeeding rates, they don't understand how women work. Breastfeeding is already idealised. Celebrities breastfeeding idealise it more, and, at the moment, not in a good way.

What all of these famous women have in common is that they never talk about breastfeeding being hard. And when the only messages we get are about the positives of nursing, we are getting only half-truths. We are being fed lies by omission. When was the last time you heard a celebrity say, 'I love breastfeeding now, but boy were those first six weeks a killer'? Or, 'We nearly didn't make it past day 10 when little Quinoa took all the skin on my nipple off, but my $200 an hour lactation consultant really helped.' Or 'Despite pumping for England, I've never been able to produce enough milk, so we top up with formula at every feed.' Ummm ... never? Correct! It's like there's some law in celebrity-land that no one is allowed to tell you the whole truth about anything to do with breastfeeding, lest they destroy their perfect earth mother image. I'm not saying every celebrity has a breastfeeding nightmare, but, surely, even with all those nannies and money for lactation consultants, they don't *all* find it easy?

The effect of these half-truths is pernicious. When Miranda Kerr posts a selfie feeding her son Flynn, her perfect breast exposed, skin flawless, smug smile intact, the message she is sending is, 'See, I can nourish my child *and* look like a smoking sex bomb.' And the message we take from it is, 'Why can't I? What's wrong with me?'

In fairness to Miranda Kerr, maybe she was just sharing what she found to be a special time with her Instagram followers. Plenty of people loved the shots and found them encouraging. But she would have done all mothers a far greater service if she also posted the occasional picture looking exhausted and grumpy at Orlando Bloom because, while she was up for the third time that night, he was still in f***ing bed.

As Susan Douglas and Meredith Michaels argue about celebrity profiles: 'The "you *can* have it all" ethos of these pieces made the rest of us feel like failures while dramatising that we could do it all if we just had the right attitude.'[72] If the women many of us see as role models only talk about breastfeeding being natural, easy and fulfilling, that's the message we will absorb. So when we find it hard, or even fail at it, where does that leave us? We haven't managed to do this most basic and essential of mothering tasks that comes naturally to these beautiful, talented women. Not only do they look amazing, they can breastfeed too. And us, stuck in our tracky bottoms, holding a bottle of formula? We're failures as women and mothers.

Unfortunately we often get sidetracked when these celebrity breastfeeding photos come out by the fools who say women shouldn't be breastfeeding in public. These people, and there are many of them, are clearly idiots. But it is annoying because we end up spending time on chat forums defending the right to breastfeed in public and to post a picture of it on Facebook, rather than talking about the photos' idealised message and what that might mean.

I don't care what Kate Middleton does with her 'royal orbs', nor do I care what Pink, Gisele or Alanis Morissette do with theirs. They are *their* breasts, and we have zero right to know whether they are breastfeeding or not. But for those celebrities who do choose to become breastfeeding role models, let's have a bit of realism about it.

It would also be wonderful if we could have a few more celebrity mums put up their hands unashamedly and say they use formula. At the moment we can count them on one hand, and with the response they get is it any wonder? Jennifer Lopez was slammed as 'miseducated' when she made public that she had chosen to formula-feed her twins.[73] Glamour model and middle-class punching bag Jordan got charities in a lather when she was featured in *OK!* bottle-feeding her three-week-old daughter.[74] (There was more to this than just anti-formula ire though. In what looked suspiciously like product placement, a large

'I don't feel guilty for bottle-feeding'

I was so excited when I found out I was pregnant because, not only am I a bottle-feeding mumma, I'm a plus size mumma too. I had read horror stories of women who were persecuted for their weight through pregnancy and their choices as a mother, and so I decided very early on that I was not going to buy into it.

Right from the start I had to mixed-feed because if I didn't my poor little man was hungry. The midwives who visited me at home were supportive of this. 'Obviously,' they told me, 'breastfeeding is best, but you don't want him going hungry.'

By six weeks my milk had dried up and I was only bottle-feeding. I didn't feel guilty; I didn't feel less of a woman or a mother. I was doing what I needed to do to make sure my boy was healthy.

And he is so healthy. He has been poorly once in his little life, a sniffle and a cough for three days, even when his father and I were sick as dogs in bed. He is at least two months ahead of most of his milestones, and has been sleeping 12 hours a night since he was about three months.

I don't feel any less bonded with my child; his smiles when he sees me prove this. Ultimately I have an extremely happy and healthy baby. He loves his bottle, he loves his veggies and fruit. Not to mention that his daddy, grandparents, aunties and uncles love to feed him as well. I have done nothing wrong as a mother – I have given my son the best I can and I wouldn't change a thing.

Kristin, Sunshine Coast, Australia, mother to Myles, 6 months

advertisement for the same formula she was using was featured next to the story, in what charities said was a breach of the WHO code on formula marketing.)

But the most over-the-top anti-formula furore to hit the headlines recently was in New Zealand, and involved All Blacks rugby star Piri Weepu. Weepu is a national hero, so when he agreed to be featured in an anti-smoking commercial for the Health Sponsorship Council it should have been a boon. Instead, a row ensued when his part in the ad was cut before it even aired. His crime? He had been filmed lovingly feeding his six-month-old baby a bottle.

Breastfeeding activist groups including La Leche League heard about the image and insisted it be cut. Their view, according to the media reports, was that the damage these two seconds of footage 'will do to breastfeeding in New Zealand will be significant'.[75] Never mind that the image was a beautiful one of a big, brawny man being actively involved in taking care of his baby. Never mind that it was two seconds long. Never mind that, as later emerged, his daughter has severe allergies, couldn't take breast milk and was on a hypoallergenic formula. Never mind that it is actually none of anyone's business how his babies are fed.[76]

The issue became a national talking point, filling the airwaves and newspaper columns for days. The most absurd comment I saw was in a television interview where a representative of the Maternity Services Council actually uttered these words to justify her condemnation of the image: 'Once the baby is born, [breastfeeding] is the most critical thing a woman can do to prevent obesity. And secondly, with the incidence of child abuse … we need to get women bonding by breastfeeding their babies.'[77] Let's put aside the questionable association with obesity, and the absurd suggestion that preventing it is the most important thing a mother can do. How about having the temerity to link child abuse to *not* breastfeeding? The ignorance and bias are simply breathtaking.

When the image of a celebrity lovingly giving his baby a bottle causes such outrage among lactivists, and those lactivists have such power that they can demand of a government agency that the image be cut, things have got out of hand.

Navigating the Breastfeeding Echo Chamber

In this chapter we've shown you how just about everything you read reinforces the flawed 'breast is best' message, from the stories you read in the newspapers, to parenting forums, to idealised images of celebrities. Given that nothing in this echo chamber is likely to change any time soon, here are some tips for navigating it:

- Don't believe every headline about a new study showing breastfeeding's benefits and formula's flaws. Find the original research yourself to look deeper – how big is the sample size, what confounders did the researchers account for, what conclusions do the researchers themselves come to, as opposed to the headline writers? The study may be top quality and legitimate – we do know, after all, that breast milk has plenty of aspects we are still learning about – but it also may not be. And remember the X factor of breastfeeding studies – the inability to separate the effects of breastfeeding from the decision to breastfeed – and how that might affect this particular paper.
- Develop a bullshit-o-meter for what you read on the internet, particularly about formula, and particularly from zealous breastfeeding sites. A lot of it is rubbish. We have listed some unbiased, trusted places for further information in the Resources section.
- Join an online or face-to-face support group for bottle-feeding families. But remember, it's not a tribal war. There is no us and them. We are all parents, and we all deserve support and respect for our decisions.
- Forget about those celebrity mums and their perfect lives. Even with their household help, nannies and professional makeup artists they have plenty of down days and motherhood challenges of their own, it's just that we don't read about those days in magazines.
- Most of all, look to your baby for guidance. Is she thriving? Is she happy? With the information overload on parenting we all now have to cope with, we can forget that the only person we should *really* be listening to is the little one in our arms. Your instincts will nearly always be right, so listen to your baby, and trust yourself. The rest is just noise.

CASE STUDY

'My breasts didn't feel like there was any milk in them. That's because there wasn't!'

Matilda was born via elective caesarean at 38 weeks and 5 days weighing 8 pounds 5 ounces. As soon as I was back in my room, the midwife insisted I try to feed her and I thought it went okay. I continued all night and *very* frequently during the day. However, Matilda was becoming more and more upset and agitated on my breast and would just scream and scream. The pain I felt was excruciating; my nipples were that sore from trying to feed round the clock that I begged the midwives to help me. One midwife brought me nipple shields, which helped a little, but Matilda was still very upset and pulling off the breast every time I tried to feed her. Another midwife tried hand-expressing me, which was so painful I cried and demanded she stop. This was day four and I started to become very concerned that something wasn't right. My breasts weren't at all tingly and they didn't feel like there was any milk in them. That's because there wasn't! I was severely anaemic and had very high blood pressure, but not one single midwife mentioned that this could affect my ability to breastfeed.

Thankfully, after me crying and feeling like a complete failure, my husband insisted we try formula. Matilda took that first bottle, drained it, then had another, almost drained it as well, then fell asleep in my arms and stayed asleep for four hours! I felt so much relief, not only physically but also emotionally. For a couple more weeks I still tried to breastfeed, mainly because I felt guilty, but she wouldn't latch on, instead she just pushed me away with her face. She was obviously wiser than I was to the fact I just wasn't producing any milk. All signs were pointing to the fact I just wasn't going to be able to feed. Matilda was three weeks old when I hung up my breasts and embraced the bottle completely. Matilda was then happily, exclusively bottle-fed from three weeks.

I think formula is the best invention ever and so does my healthy, thriving 28-month-old daughter, who is in the 97th percentile for height.

continued

continued from previous page

Formula allowed me to feed my growing child when my body failed. I am so thrilled with how well formula nourished my first child that I will be feeding my second child formula as well at some point too. That may be from seven days old or seven months old – at this point I'm not sure. We'll see how breastfeeding goes.

I feel very protective now of mothers who choose to use formula or had to use formula, and very thankful to the mummies who supported me and assured me formula was fine.

Kate, Sydney, mother to Matilda, 28 months, and
8 months pregnant with baby number 2

4 Guilt, pressure and support

Along with baby wipes, hand sanitiser and Facebook, guilt is the modern mother's constant companion. It's a friend, a foe, a fricking pain in the arse. 'Mother's ruin' used to be what people called gin. These days what ruins motherhood isn't gin (how could a G and T ever be anything but helpful?): it's guilt.

Here are some things I feel guilty about, two years into the long march of motherhood: working; not working; using frozen fish fingers instead of making my own; sending my daughter out in clean but stained, unironed clothes; not knowing as much about current affairs as I used to; the relief I feel when my daughter goes to day care and my time is my own; having a glass of wine most nights; not exercising enough; struggling to find dinner conversation topics with a 2-year-old; not being that fun mum who has a craft box and endless ideas; making birthday cakes from packet mix instead of from scratch; enjoying a champagne or three at a friend's wedding when I was unknowingly pregnant; my lack of sex drive; my tired grumpiness; not paying my husband enough attention; not paying my friends enough attention; not paying my daughter enough attention. You get the picture. Your own guilt list may have similar themes.

But the biggest guilt kicker for most mums is using formula. Guilt, a sense of failure, uncertainty and being worried about what the midwife might say are all emotions common to mothers who bottle-feed.[1] What causes this guilt? Why do we feel it about feeding more than anything else when a majority of us use formula at some stage? What role do midwives and health professionals have to play? What effect does it have on our mental health? And how can we get rid of it? These are the issues we'll be looking at in this chapter. We'll start by examining the pressure that comes from those people who have such fleeting but influential roles in our lives as parents – the midwives, nurses, doctors and health visitors who care for us when we have a baby.

The role of health professionals

We look to health professionals to be superheroes in our hour of need. So many do a fantastic job with what must, quite a lot of the time, feel like a thankless task. However, when it comes to feeding, many women complain about the guilt and pressure to breastfeed they feel from nurses, doctors, midwives and health visitors. In this section we'll look at this pressure. We'll also discuss the role of the Baby Friendly Initiative, how the promotion of breastfeeding has stifled health professionals from giving information about formula-feeding, and what needs to change to better support both breastfeeding *and* bottle-feeding parents.

CASE STUDY

Mums' experiences of health professionals

I asked Bottle Babies members on Facebook about the pressure and support they had received from health staff.[2] Their range of experiences show how inconsistent, and often 'pushy', the approach to breastfeeding and bottle-feeding is.

There was a lot of pressure for me to breastfeed, and because Bub wouldn't latch she developed hypoglycaemia while in hospital. No one mentioned a bottle to me, but they continued to try to force the baby to my breast. I kept trying for six weeks, with help from the 'support' people, on a few occasions being left in tears after I was told I wasn't 'trying hard enough to feed baby', even though she still refused to latch.

Nerissa

There is no support in hospital for bottle-feeding. I had to sign a form to say I understood breast was best and the risks involved in bottle-feeding.

No advice on amount of formula, sterilising, etc. Some midwives were happy and supported my decision but others totally ignored the fact. I think it is ridiculous they cannot support a mother either way.

Kaylene

I am disturbed that child health nurses cannot advise on bottle-feeding. Surely making sure the baby is fed is part of their job?

Sue

Breastfeeding was the only way that the hospital promoted feeding your child (even at antenatal classes), so when I did not produce any milk they tried everything to get me to feed on the breast. They pulled and prodded me until my nipples were so sore and bleeding. I was crying and felt like a failure to my child, then my obstetrician arrived and took one look at me and said, 'Feed your child with a bottle, he will not care and he will love you no matter how you feed him.' I could have jumped off the bed and cuddled her.

Elita

I was unable to get my daughter to latch and spent a whole shift with one of the hospital lactation consultants who was amazing and guided me in the end into combination feeding, i.e. expressed milk and formula feeds. She was very supportive and encouraging and made me feel that although I wasn't able to directly feed my daughter I was doing the best that my body would allow. In contrast, a different lactation consultant at the same hospital told me when my daughter was four weeks old that as she had always had a bottle she would never bond with me and I was a complete stranger to my baby. Understandably, I cried for 24 hours thinking that I had failed my daughter.

Janine

The fine line between support and pressure

Midwives and health visitors are in a difficult situation when it comes to feeding – on the one hand they are supposed to promote and encourage breastfeeding; on the other, they need to support all mothers, regardless of feeding choice.[3] It's a dilemma, and at the moment the balance is not right – some women feel pushed by midwives to breastfeed, but not always sufficiently supported in both breastfeeding and the alternatives. In the 2013 report by the Care Quality Commission, 41% of women surveyed felt inadequately supported in the process of breastfeeding, and one in six women who talked about feeding said they felt overwhelmed by the pressure to breastfeed, and this made them feel isolated and guilty.[4]

While it would be very rare for a midwife to explicitly say 'you must breastfeed', as one mother put it to Australian researchers:

> ❝The professionals make you feel that you should continue breastfeeding at all costs. You can tell they don't want you to bottle-feed. They never even mention bottles – you have to kind of ask, and sometimes even when you do ask about bottles they don't answer your questions – they just keep saying, 'Oh no, you can do it.'[5]❞

This pressure to 'just keep going' is one that has a personal ring for me. Despite telling every single health worker I came into contact with when my daughter was born about my breast reduction – one of the biggest physical impediments to breastfeeding – I was repeatedly told to just keep on feeding, and that my milk would eventually come in. It took until day six, after my baby had lost 13% of her birthweight, for a health visitor to suggest I top up with formula. What the 12 or more health professionals I had previously come into contact with, both ante- and postnatally, should have been discussing was the very strong likelihood that I would never produce enough milk to feed my baby, and how to manage that so that she could get the benefits of the breast milk I could produce while getting the calories she needed from elsewhere.

Looking back on it now, I feel failed by those midwives who pressured me to continue breastfeeding exclusively, despite my obvious and predictable lack of milk. I would have liked to learn about supplemental nursing systems – they weren't mentioned. I would have liked a nurse to properly listen to me rather than just rush to her next patient – I felt like I was just a box to be ticked. But most of all I would have liked for my baby not to cry with hunger for six days straight with me not knowing what to do other than 'just keep going' because that was what every single health professional told me to do.

I asked Janet Fyle, a practising midwife and professional policy adviser at the Royal College of Midwives, if she and her colleagues sometimes feel in a difficult position when it comes to how to deal with baby feeding. She told me no – as professionals, their role is clear.

"If one is a professional and you've been asked to care for people who come to you with different values and beliefs, you need to do so in a manner that doesn't bring to the table your own views. So, for example . . . the woman who says, 'I don't want to breastfeed, I don't like it.' Maybe the midwife might be interested to find out why the woman doesn't want to, maybe to offer other types of help, though not to persuade her not to bottle-feed. You cannot persuade a woman to do something that she has chosen not to do. The best thing you can do in that situation is to make sure that she does so properly.[6]**"**

While Ms Fyle's position sounds fine in theory, in practice we know that so often it just doesn't work like this. Many women who choose formula, either exclusively or in combination with the breast, feel judged and dismissed by health professionals. That has the effect of breeding resentment and a lack of trust[7] – one survey of British mums who had used formula found that a quarter were worried about what the midwife or health visitor would say.[8] Some mothers have even admitted to researchers that they lie to midwives and health visitors about using formula, because they don't want to be subjected to judgement.

One major reason for this pressure is that guidelines and recommendations around promoting breastfeeding are often misinterpreted, or applied too rigidly.[9]

The Baby Friendly Initiative

The most highly regarded guidelines are those established for UNICEF's Baby Friendly Initiative. It's a programme designed to increase breastfeeding rates by giving better support for women antenatally, and then right from the moment they deliver in hospital. In order to get Baby Friendly accreditation, hospitals need to follow the 'Ten Steps to Successful Breastfeeding'.

The Baby Friendly Initiative's 'Ten Steps to Successful Breastfeeding'

1. Develop a breastfeeding policy: have a written breastfeeding policy that is routinely communicated to all healthcare staff.

2. Ensure staff receive training: train all healthcare staff in skills necessary to implement this policy.

3. Provide antenatal information: inform all pregnant women about the benefits and management of breastfeeding.

4. Help initiate breastfeeding: place babies in skin-to-skin contact with their mothers immediately following birth for at least an hour and encourage mothers to recognise when their babies are ready to breastfeed, offering help if needed.

5. Teach breastfeeding: show mothers how to breastfeed and how to maintain lactation even if they should be separated from their infants.

6. Avoid supplementation: give newborn infants no food or drink other than breast milk, unless medically indicated.

7. Practice rooming-in: allow mothers and infants to remain together 24 hours a day.

8. Encourage breastfeeding on demand.

9. Give no artificial teats or dummies to breastfeeding infants.

10. Provide access to support groups: foster the establishment of breastfeeding support and refer mothers on discharge from the facility.[10]

At the time of writing, nearly a third of all UK hospitals were Baby Friendly accredited and 55% were working towards accreditation.[11] In Australia, around 20% of maternity facilities were Baby Friendly.[12] The programme has influenced the entire maternity sector; midwives at non-accredited hospitals often follow the Ten Steps informally.

However, in giving midwives and maternity nurses guidelines for promoting breastfeeding, the natural human tendency to follow rules to the letter sometimes kicks in. For example, a study of Australian women's feeding decisions found that '[Maternity] policies and practices do not acknowledge the need for individualised care ... This is exemplified in the ten steps to successful breastfeeding, which are often applied rigidly, and do not encompass the need for sensitive care or the need to address women's emotional needs.'[13] They added that applying global initiatives such as the BFI in a '"top down" bureaucratic manner' can result in some women feeling pressure to breastfeed.

It's a view that Janet Fyle, adviser to the Royal College of Midwives, seemed to agree with. 'The BFI has worked in that you get midwives to engage in the discussion about breastfeeding and its benefits, but it should not be used to beat women about the head,' she said.

While describing the Baby Friendly accreditation as 'brilliant', Ms Fyle also says she reminds her colleagues that, 'Midwives are not agents of Baby Friendly . . . they are employed by the NHS, and [we] have to focus on who the NHS's clients and patients are.'

It's a refreshing view, as one of the biggest criticisms of the Baby Friendly programme, and maternity units' approaches to breastfeeding more generally, is that they focus so much on breastfeeding but little on the relationship between a mother and her baby, or on the bigger picture of the birth experience and adjusting to a new life with a little one.[14] As parents, we know that feeding can't be isolated from the rest of the new baby whirlwind, but that is how it has often been treated – as a medical problem to be addressed in isolation.

Despite these problems, the Baby Friendly standards are considered to be the 'gold standard' as far as promoting breastfeeding is concerned. Yet, there are also legitimate questions about how successful they have been. For example, although BF hospitals have increased the number of women who start breastfeeding in hospital, a large study of low-income mums in Britain found that, four weeks in, those mums who had given birth in BF facilities were no more likely to be breastfeeding than mums who had delivered at unaccredited hospitals.[15]

The welcome winds of change

In good news, it seems that those who run the Baby Friendly Initiative are becoming aware of some of its shortcomings. In 2013 in the UK, the BFI brought in new standards that recognise there needs to be a greater focus on the holistic care of mothers and babies, on building the relationship of a mother and baby beyond feeding, and on a mother's own feelings and needs.[16] This is a welcome change, and it shows that the medical profession is listening to mothers who have long complained of not having their needs met, and pragmatic experts who have argued that: 'A woman-centred advocate who supports a mother's own decisions and helps her to feel positive about herself and her role as a mother would be more effective than a breastfeeding-centred advocate.'[17]

What effect these changes to the BFI will have in practice remains to be seen, but in order to implement a more sensitive approach to mothers and babies it could be argued that what is needed in addition to a change in mindset is more midwife time, and in a hospital context midwife time means money. Without a significant investment by governments in improving midwife and doctor care, it's hard to imagine that the experience of new mothers and their babies will change significantly.

Sasha says:

The reality of working in a busy NHS delivery suite and postnatal ward is that it is hectic, stressful and demanding. Midwives, nurses, doctors and healthcare assistants are often stretched to the limits of their capacity, running from one task to the next, understandably prioritising the sickest and neediest patients and often, in my own experience, hugely aware of what more they would like to be doing for their patients if they had the time and capacity.

In contrast, what a new mum struggling to feed needs is time, patience, focus and understanding. And, of course, an experienced professional around and available at the time you are actually feeding your baby. It's not very helpful to be in the middle of being shown how to get a good latch by a midwife when the emergency call bell goes and she has to run, or the junior doctor's bleep goes off three times in a minute.

The ideal is to have specialist breastfeeding consultants available on the postnatal ward and these brilliant people do exist, although not in great enough numbers. But in the modern world when women are discharged as soon as humanly possible after their delivery, it is often just not feasible to have more than one feed observed by a breastfeeding consultant. In our mothers' day, women would spend a week in hospital after their first delivery, to recover *and* to learn how to feed. Now we find ourselves back in our own living rooms 12 hours after delivery, with a tiny screaming infant to feed and a hazy blur of breastfeeding advice in our minds, but very limited know-how. It's little wonder most of us struggle to get it right.

Lack of support and information for formula-feeding families

Another major effect of the vigorous promotion of breastfeeding at maternity facilities is the shameful lack of support and information for formula-feeding families. Multiple studies and anecdotal evidence show that there is a perception that midwives 'aren't allowed' to talk about formula and that parents are left to figure out how to formula-feed themselves, both in hospitals and after discharge.[18] It continues a conspiracy of silence about formula-feeding that begins antenatally, as though if medical professionals don't talk about it, it will just go away. The effect of this is that an alarming number of families are preparing, handling and giving bottles incorrectly. As the authors of a systematic review into mothers' experiences of bottle-feeding warned: 'Inadequate information and support for mothers who decide to bottle-feed may put the health of their babies at risk.'[19]

I know this only too well from experience. When our third health visitor finally advised my husband and me to top our daughter up with formula, she didn't talk about any aspects of formula-feeding, she just told us to do what it said on the tin. Unfortunately, my husband misread the instructions, and for the first couple of days we gave her formula that was watered down by two-thirds. (Imagine the ear-bashing he got when I discovered our error!)

We learned about sterilising from our friends who gave us their steriliser. I looked at websites, which gave conflicting advice about how to make up feeds, and got no advice whatsoever about how to read my baby's cues for when she had had enough, or the importance of feeding sensitively to promote bonding and attachment. In short, it was a shambles – a mishmash of ad hoc unprofessional advice that we bumbled our way through, and that potentially put our daughter's health at risk. Your own experience has likely been similar. This is not good enough. Mothers and babies deserve better. We *need* better.

Some midwives themselves are under the mistaken belief that under Baby Friendly guidelines they aren't allowed to talk about formula at all, including demonstrating how to use a bottle.[20] *This is not true.* In the UK, both national guidelines and Baby Friendly guidelines say that a mother who has chosen to bottle-feed *should be instructed in how to make up a bottle*.[21] They also say that, although groups of women aren't allowed to be taught about bottles in antenatal classes, if women request it, they can be verbally taught about bottles one on one before the baby is born. (The guidelines prohibit an actual demonstration until *after* the birth.)

However, in practice we know that this just doesn't happen. In a survey of British formula-feeding mums done in 2005, only 45% said they had received information about formula from midwives, and only 20% from health visitors.[22] (Some received it from both.) Worryingly, more than half said they had received no information at all about formula-feeding. Another study found that many mums don't think it's possible to overfeed babies and don't fully understand how to read babies' hunger cues.[23] This is also a big worry, as these are believed to be factors in the higher rates of obesity among formula-fed babies.

The midwives don't know

One big hurdle is that midwives themselves often have little knowledge of formula and best practice for making and storing it. As an example, only 18% of midwives surveyed by a market research company in 2008 knew there was a difference between different types of formula milk.[24] As one midwife told a researcher, 'I think there's a lack of adequate knowledge about it, about the milk. I mean we can give a little bit but I couldn't sit and talk more than two or three minutes about formula-feeds because I just don't have that information. Whereas breastfeeding, I could sit and talk all day about it.'[25]

While breastfeeding is extensively discussed in midwifery curricula (which is obviously needed and appropriate), formula-feeding education is patchy. Learning about formula is in the curriculum, but it is up to each university to determine how much or how little is taught. In practice, that can mean hundreds of midwives every year graduating with very little knowledge of bottle-feeding.

Even if health professionals want to learn about formula after they graduate, they face the same problems we do as mums – there is very little unbiased information for them to refer to. When the majority of mothers use formula at some stage, and 20% of mothers use it from birth, this is a huge and serious knowledge gap. As one British researcher put it: 'there are national guidelines that support a policy of health professionals giving mothers who formula-feed the information they require. Health professionals who do not do this are failing in their professional duty.'[26]

The new standards for the Baby Friendly Initiative in the UK have recognised that bottle-feeding families need better support. Criteria for assessment now specifically state that staff should encourage loving relationships between parents and babies during bottle-feeding, encourage the first bottle-feed to be skin to skin and teach how to respond to babies' cues, and that health visitors should provide information for formula-feeding mothers.

This is a good first step, and let's hope it is implemented well. But we need to do more to promote safe, loving bottle-feeding and to ensure that mothers don't feel judged if they are not breastfeeding exclusively.

'No health workers had the time or patience to help us breastfeed'

CASE STUDY

I desperately wanted to breastfeed and shamefully admit now that I had judged other mothers who didn't, as I had been totally sucked in by the propaganda. I also wanted, very much, to feed my son for free – we are not a rich family in financial terms.

The only feeding support we had while we were in hospital was midwives hurriedly coming in and manhandling me to get my son to feed rather than sitting with me and giving me the time I needed. I had to express into a cup and feed him with a syringe because nobody had the time or patience to deal with us. On our discharge from hospital they said that we were feeding well, but I wouldn't have put it that way. A call to the breastfeeding helpline just reiterated the propaganda, telling me not to turn to the bottle, and to wait for specialist help.

continued

continued from previous page

When a lactation support worker came twice in one day, even with her 10 years of experience it took half an hour to get my son feeding properly each time. But when she left I couldn't get it to work, so I felt that expressing was my only option, and my milk wasn't coming in. Once my son latched on he would just fall asleep and wouldn't feed no matter what I did.

I was drifting into a very dark place – my postnatal depression was beginning to kick in and, unbeknownst to me at the time, my postnatal PTSD due to a traumatic birth experience.

I am so glad that I found it within myself to ask my husband if he would support me if I said I couldn't breastfeed and he thankfully did, and on day three we turned to formula. Thank God for formula! I began bonding with my baby at last. After his first feed from the bottle his eyes opened wide – it was a wonderful thing to see. I knew I was doing the best for him.

Support for feeding was dropped from that point and we had to find our own way. Guilt was laid on at every opportunity by healthcare professionals. I still feel very angry about that time. I no longer feel guilty about feeding formula to my son, although I do feel guilty about the time I wasted feeling guilty because of all the pressure and propaganda around me.

Gemm, Cornwall, mother to Jago, 10 months

What bottle-feeding families need

Midwives, other hospital staff and health visitors need to be better trained not only in the 'how tos' of formula-feeding but in how to discuss formula-feeding without coming across as being judgemental. Many midwives already do this beautifully; others don't. Given the large numbers of bottle-feeding women that midwives and health visitors care for, this needs to be tackled in a head-on manner, as a matter of urgency.

Under current guidelines, information about bottle-feeding is supposed to be given to women by health professionals when they ask for it. Given that most British women are still attempting to breastfeed exclusively at discharge, but by the end of the first week of their baby's life half will have introduced some formula, the responsible, prudent course of action is to give *all* mothers the NHS information booklet on bottle-feeding when they leave hospital, regardless of their stated feeding intention.

The argument raised against this is that it promotes using formula. Perhaps for a few women it will, but the reality is that large numbers of women are choosing formula anyway – 73% of six-week-old British babies have been given at least one formula bottle despite the concerted, decades-long campaign against it. It's time to accept that, while the fight to protect and encourage breastfeeding must go on, doing so by imposing a conspiracy of silence and ignorance around formula-feeding has failed. To use a well-worn phrase, we must move to 'harm minimisation' and provide readily accessible information to families to try to prevent the overfeeding, diarrhoea, malnutrition, ear infections and insensitive feeding that can result when families are left to figure out bottle-feeding for themselves. Families want this information. Health professionals are the people who should be delivering it.

At the time of writing, trials are currently under way in both the UK and Australia to test what effect one-to-one bottle-feeding support might have in promoting healthy growth patterns (i.e. reducing obesity) in formula-fed babies.[27] Wouldn't it be great if all parents could have access to a bottle-feeding counsellor in the same way breastfeeding mums can drop in to a baby cafe or request a free breastfeeding counsellor? Bottle-feeding usually doesn't present the various ongoing and diverse challenges that breastfeeding does, but one-to-one education to learn the important skills of sterilising, preparation, reading babies' cues, how to bottle-feed to promote bonding, and awareness of possible problems would be welcomed with open arms by parents who currently feel completely in the dark. It would also benefit the health system, which would likely see fewer babies presenting with problems caused by poor bottle preparation.

> ## Sasha says:
>
> We cannot focus on the breastfeeding mums and put all our energy and attention into promoting breastfeeding, but then consign them to the 'failed' bin if they can't or don't want to breastfeed. The reality cannot be this black and white. There are breastfeeders and formula-feeders and every shade in between, and each of them needs a different, personalised combination of support and advice. If this individualised approach could begin prior to delivery, it would be even better.

In addition to access to a bottle-feeding counsellor (or a breastfeeding counsellor who has more than a passing knowledge of formula), how about a 24-hour independent bottle-feeding helpline, similar to breastfeeding helplines? Formula companies provide these services, but we need unbiased sources of help and information.

The Fearless Formula Feeder Suzanne Barston wants a new initiative to work alongside the Baby Friendly Initiative in the US where she lives. She calls it the Family Friendly Hospital Initiative.

'Our main goal is to ensure that, with so many hospitals here in the US adopting the BFI standards, mothers are not neglected or harassed emotionally or physically in the process of trying to raise breastfeeding rates,' she told me. The main planks include:

- ensuring that all mothers-to-be and their partners receive fact-based, non-emotional literature about the pros and cons of *all* feeding methods before they give birth
- obliging hospitals to give true autonomy to mothers, not only in their birth plans, as is currently the norm, but in feeding too – this means instruction in formula use as well as respecting a woman's intention to breastfeed
- allowing antenatal classes and postnatal groups to discuss bottle-feeding, and providing groups that focus on maternal health rather than on just breastfeeding
- providing a certification for midwives, lactation consultants and nurses who wish to provide the women they are caring for with a more holistic approach to whatever type of feeding they decide is right for them, including giving bottle-feeding support.

They are all excellent ideas, and Suzanne and her team of volunteers are committed to making them a reality.

In order to improve the health of bottle-fed babies, and improve the mental health and welfare of their parents, we as a society, and medical professionals in particular, urgently need to take a more individualised approach to caring for mothers and babies. We need to change the 'one-size-fits-all' mentality of current breastfeeding promotion and see feeding as part of a much wider and more complicated parenting relationship, one where bottle-feeding is also respected and valued. Midwives, nurses, doctors and lactation consultants should be at the vanguard of this.

'Mother's ruin'

"Guilt: a feeling of having committed wrong or failed in an obligation.**"**
Oxford English Dictionary[40]

Guilt about bottle-feeding has become so common that psychologists have observed that it has become the 'normal' and 'natural' response for formula-feeding mothers.[41] Think about it. Have any of your mother friends ever told you they've changed to formula without giving a long justification as to why? How many times have you, when you've pulled out a bottle, felt the need to list the problems you had breastfeeding and tell people how hard you tried before you eventually 'gave up'?

How did we get to this crazy situation, where the way that the majority of us at least partially feed our babies comes with an obligatory side serving of guilt? 'Well, because "breast is best", and if you're not doing the best for your baby, then you feel guilty,' is the obvious reply. And that is entirely correct … as a first answer. But dig a little deeper and you find there are a number of powerful cultural forces and underlying assumptions about babies, motherhood and feeding that underpin it. They include the overplayed benefits of breast milk, an intensive mothering culture and our modern obsession with minimising risk, which have all led to feeding becoming a moral issue rather than a practical one. Let's examine those in more detail now.

Postnatal depression and breastfeeding pressure[28]

'The pressure to breastfeed was 100% behind my postnatal depression,' says Emma Shepherd, a mum of two from Bristol. Having successfully breastfed her first son for 10 months, she assumed she would have no trouble feeding her second. But when George developed serious reflux she hit a snag. Doctors and nurses erroneously told her that if he was having bottles they could have given him medication, but because he was being breastfed there was nothing they could do. Emma says when she floated the idea of bottle-feeding she was told the most important thing she could do was breastfeed George, and to keep going, so she did.

After three months of tortured feedings, sleep deprivation and guilt, Emma was diagnosed with postnatal depression. 'If I'd switched to bottles at the start, or if I'd been given more of a choice, I don't believe I would have developed it. To this day, eight years later, I feel guilty about not questioning the doctors further,'[29] she says. Emma is not alone.

Around 10% to 15% of all new mothers develop postnatal depression (PND) or postnatal anxiety (PNA).[30] The prevailing view is that women who don't breastfeed are more at risk of developing depression, and this is backed up by research. Much clinical attention has been spent on trying to find ways to enable depressed mothers to continue breastfeeding. But new evidence is starting to emerge that suggests that, rather than weaning from the breast being a side effect of PND and PNA, the pressure to breastfeed could actually be a *contributing factor* in women developing postnatal mood disorders in the first place.

An Australian study conducted by the country's leading mental health charity, Beyond Blue, questioned 42 women with PND or PNA about their experience during pregnancy and the first six months after delivery. More than 95% spontaneously said that difficulties with breastfeeding and the resulting guilt and sadness had contributed to their illness.[31]

'The women talked about the portrayal of perfect mothers in the media who are all breastfeeding, and how it made them feel like a failure when they were having troubles,' says Dr Nicole Highet, who led the study. 'They also mentioned the staff at hospitals who just say to "keep going, keep going" – they called them the breastfeeding Nazis – but were actually not that helpful at sorting out problems with feeding.'[32]

A small Norwegian study, published in 2012, produced similar results.[33] Silje Marie Haga, who led the Norwegian research, said that all the mothers in her study viewed breastfeeding as being synonymous with being a good mother.

'That's why it was very stressful when they didn't succeed because they see it as stopping them from being a good enough mum. And when women struggle with breastfeeding they are more likely to become isolated because they don't want to go outside if they don't feel comfortable, so you can see a snowballing effect on depression and anxiety because social support is so important.'[34]

A number of PND counsellors have confirmed anecdotally that the pressure to be a perfect mother, most strongly exemplified by breastfeeding, is increasing, and having an increasingly detrimental effect on mothers' mental health.

'I see many women in my practice for whom this is an issue,' says Liz Wise, a specialist PND counsellor in Surrey. 'Over the past 15 years the need to be a perfect mother is becoming more and more prevalent, and breastfeeding plays a huge role in the image of the perfect mother.'[35]

'At least 70% of the clients I work with talk about issues around breastfeeding,' says Rima Sidhpara, a Leicester-based psychotherapist. 'I think it is unrecognised in the literature, and it's important that it is highlighted.'[36]

The relationship between breastfeeding and PNA/PND is a complex one. For some depressed mothers, breastfeeding is a lifeline, the only positive moments in their day. On the other hand, depressed women who are struggling to breastfeed can feel like failures, which can further compound their symptoms. But the idea, suggested by the Australian and Norwegian research, that the pressure to breastfeed could be a trigger for postnatal mood disorders is a new one.

Kate Kripke, a PND counsellor who blogs for PostPartumProgress.com, says, 'It's hard to say whether the challenges in breastfeeding are a cause of mom's distress or a result of it. And, of course, there are also many women who I work with who love to breastfeed, and in these situations the breastfeeding is the one thing that these moms hold on to.'[37]

Treating PND and PNA is important not only for mothers but also for babies. The children of depressed and anxious mothers tend to score lower on emotional and social tests than children of healthy mothers,[38] and they can be less securely attached[39] as toddlers.

While work continues into researching the physical causes of both postnatal mood disorders and difficulty lactating, it seems obvious that the pressure to breastfeed – whether perceived external pressure or a mother's own expectations of herself – is playing a role.

Kate Kripke says it's important that mothers know that their relationship with their baby is far more important than how they feed them. 'Breast milk is best, but babies need their mums much more than the breast milk. If the anxiety around breastfeeding means a mother is not as attuned to her baby because she's worried about the feeding, then that's problematic. Forget about the breast milk. The attachment far outweighs the importance of breast milk.'

'Breast is best'

We've already looked in Chapter 2 at how the benefits of breast milk in the developed world have been overplayed. We demonstrated that contrary to what alarmist websites and extreme breastfeeding advocates will tell you, it *is* possible to raise a happy, healthy, smart and wonderfully bonded baby who is formula-fed. Then, in Chapter 3, we saw how these exaggerated benefits have been reinforced by the Breastfeeding Echo Chamber, where they have been repeated so many times that they have become unassailable 'facts' we can't escape.

Because breastfeeding is portrayed as being vastly superior to bottle-feeding, it is positioned as the only viable 'choice' for a responsible mother. And in our modern world, mothers must *always* make the best choice for their babies regardless of the cost to themselves – this is part of our all-pervading culture of *intensive mothering*.

Intensive mothering

Ask your mum what she thinks the differences are between being a mother 30 years ago and now.

I asked mine, and her answer was pretty eye-opening.

❝I think the pressure on modern mothers to be the perfect mother is enormous. It really makes it tough, but a lot of times it's self-imposed. The mothers themselves think they should be able to do it all. And I think maybe it's because lots of you don't have the same support network because families are so spread out, that you feel really intensely involved in looking after this baby. Perhaps the older age of mothers is a factor. And families are smaller, so that increases the intensity. There's also so much advisory material about the 'right' way to do stuff. How to handle your baby, how to position your baby, how to *handle your relationship with your partner. It's often done with scientific backup, but so much of it is contradictory. A lot of it is very helpful but it comes at a cost – I think it probably makes it harder for any instinctive mothering.*"

And there it is: my mother has basically summed up in 10 sentences what hundreds of academics and authors have expended thousands of pages saying – modern mothering is one big pressure cooker.

Somehow, over the last generation, being a mother has stopped being something that you just got on with. It has become a double-full-time occupation, which we must study for, sacrifice for, work ourselves to the bone for.

This 'intensive mothering' has become a recognised sociological phenomenon, the dominant parenting discourse of our time, and one that all of us, whether we recognise it or not, will fall in line with to a greater or lesser extent. It's dominated by five major tenets: that women are naturally better at parenting than men; that parenting should be fulfilling; that children need to be cognitively stimulated by parents; that mothering is hard, 'the hardest job in the world'; and that parents should prioritise their children's needs over their own.[42]

Do any of those sound familiar? Have you ever dismissed your male partner because he's just not changing that nappy right and only *you* can do it properly? (Me.) Ever sat fruitlessly trying to get a 15-month-old to build blocks when they'd rather eat them, because you've been told it 'helps their development'? (Erm, me again.) How about buying organic mince for your little one's specially made no-salt meatballs, while you get by on the regular kind mixed with bottled spaghetti sauce. (Yep.) Those might just seem like normal things to do, but they are actually all expressions of intensive mothering, and the fact we think they are normal shows how much the ideology has come to dominate middle-class Western life.

Intensive mothering goes hand in hand with the idea of a child being precious, and childhood being something to be protected. Believe it or not, parenthood and childhood have not always been like this. In centuries past, parents used to send their children away to be raised by wet nurses. Children were beaten into submission, and even sedated for misbehaviour. In many societies, across many centuries, children were viewed as either workers, or burdens until they were old enough to become workers. Childhood was not a special time. The notion that parents, especially mothers, need to be a constant loving, stimulating presence is something relatively new, which has grown out of the rise of the Western middle class over the last few centuries, and particularly in the last 50 years.[43] I'm not saying that those old ways of raising children were good – I see them as horrible. But we need to realise that everything, including parenting, goes through fashions and fads, and our own view of what is appropriate and normal can't be separated from those wider influences.

At the moment, we are in a period where we believe that being a good parent means being an informed, attentive, intensive parent. It's why Amazon lists over 70,000 titles if you search under 'parenting books', and why taking your baby to do yoga, or to hear French nursery rhymes, or to a massage class, or to special baby classical music concerts are all normal. It's the reason why both working and stay-at-home mothers spend on average 6.5 hours more per week actively engaging with their children than they did 30 years ago, usually because they are now folding their own personal leisure time in with their children's activities.[44] The authors Susan J. Douglas and Meredith W. Michaels call it ' "the new momism": the insistence that no woman is truly complete or fulfilled until she has kids, that women remain the best primary caretaker of children, and that to be a remotely decent mother, a woman has to devote her entire physical, psychological, emotional and intellectual being, 24/7, to her children'.[45]

Breastfeeding fits in perfectly with the intensive mothering and 'new momism' ideologies: it is something only women can do; it is billed as being wonderfully fulfilling for a mother; it is promoted as stimulating babies' brains; it's often hard, at least in the beginning; and it most certainly prioritises a baby's needs above our own. Bottle-feeding is portrayed as being the exact opposite: selfish; risky to babies' brain development; not promoting a special bond between mother and baby; and the easy way out. Is it any wonder that parents who deviate from the dominant intensive motherhood ideology and use formula feel guilty? This one act is so much more than simply choosing a different form of nourishment – it is breaking all the cardinal rules of modern mothering.

'I was being extremely tough on myself'

I had a c-section with Evie as I had pre-eclampsia and couldn't be induced. As soon as she was born she latched on and I breastfed her. But for some reason she had trouble feeding after that initial feed. The midwives were very supportive and we tried lots of different positions to get her to latch on again. For about a week I tried breastfeeding alongside bottle-feeding, but got progressively more frustrated, tired and demoralised. I felt like other mums were going to judge me, as though I was an outsider to all these wonderful breastfeeding mothers, and letting Evie down by not giving her the best. As well as struggling over feeding, I was also recovering from a traumatic c-section and losing 1.5 litres of blood. I was still expressing milk for her, so she was getting some breast milk for about six weeks. I didn't get any negative opinions from anyone about using formula, even the health visitors and midwives were fairly supportive, but I was being extremely tough on myself. I finally got to the point where I realised it was just pressure that I was putting on myself and it was far more important that Evie was happy, well fed and sleeping than me striving for this idealistic picture of motherhood. She needed me to be a relaxed, calm mum, not one who was worn out and crying every time I tried to feed her. So, after about six weeks, I finally accepted that I would be exclusively formula-feeding her and we settled into a good routine. I can now say that I am so glad I decided to bottle-feed Evie. We have a very close relationship and there has never been any question of us not having a strong bond.

Deborah, London, mother to Evie, 9 months

Minimise every risk

The intensive mothering ideology works in partnership with the risk culture that our modern Western lives sit within. As newspapers are so fond of telling us, in the early twenty-first century, untold dangers are always lurking just around the corner: from paedophiles to stray rusty nails, internet bullies to undercooked chicken. It's a minefield.

Someone who thinks about this a lot is Lenore Skenazy, the author and founder of the Free-Range Kids movement and blog. Lenore has made it her mission in life to try to get parents to chill out, to trust their kids more and to lay off the helicopter intensity and risk-aversion. When we chatted over Skype from her home in New York she told me that risk culture has come to dominate how we think about our kids.

> **"**As parents, we've decided to see everything through the lens of risk. We're all thinking like lawyers, partly because of our litigious society. And what we have done as a society is lose the understanding of the difference between risk, which is inherent in everything, and risky. And when you start seeing everything as risky, then nothing is ever safe enough.**"**

When risk culture meets intensive mothering, the end result is that one of a mother's main roles has become minimising every possible risk to her child, no matter how small.[46] You're pregnant and you just got served a slightly runny poached egg? Better send it back to the kitchen because there's a one in a million chance it contains listeria. You've read that lots of kids have peanut allergies these days? No peanut butter for your little treasure until they're 2, even though there's no history of peanut allergies in the family. Your kid might fall off the climbing frame at the playground and hit her head? Stay within arm's reach of her at all times, and better still, make her wear a helmet. (Don't laugh – there are parents at my local park who actually do this.) Of course, there's now a risk she could end up a quivering, cowardly pile of jelly because she's never been allowed to have anything bad happen to her in her life, but, oh well. At least she's *safe*.

The general and parenting media fan the flames of our paranoia with endless articles such as '8 foods your toddler could be allergic to',[47] and 'A surprising risk for toddlers on playground slides'.[48] Forget the fact that most toddlers aren't allergic to foods, and the vast majority of children go down slides without terrible accidents, the seed of the fear has been planted. And if you've been warned of the risks and something bad *does* happen, it will not be a simple accident – it will be *your fault* that you didn't manage out that risk.

The power of risk has been taken to heart by the breastfeeding lobby. You'll notice that as often now as we are told about the *benefits* of breastfeeding, we are told about the *risks* of formula-feeding. The strategy was hit upon by a canny breastfeeding advocate, Dianne Wiessinger, in an essay published in 1996 called 'Watch your language'. In it, she urges other advocates to change the way they speak about breastfeeding and formula-feeding, because using the stick of 'risk' is, she argues, more powerful than the carrot of 'benefit'. Her thoughts are worth quoting at length to show the way our emotions have been deliberately manipulated and preyed upon by zealous lactivists.[49]

66*Are you the best possible parent? Is your home life ideal? Do you provide optimal meals? Of course not. Those are admirable goals, not minimum standards. Let's rephrase. Is your parenting inadequate? Is your home life subnormal? Do you provide deficient meals? Now it hurts. You may not expect to be far above normal, but you certainly don't want to be below normal . . . The truth is, breastfeeding is nothing more than normal. Artificial feeding, which is neither the same nor superior, is therefore deficient, incomplete, and inferior. Those are difficult words, but they have an appropriate place in our vocabulary . . . Because breastfeeding is the biological norm, breastfed babies are not 'healthier'; artificially-fed babies are ill more often and more seriously. Breastfed babies do not 'smell better'; artificial feeding results in an abnormal and unpleasant odor that reflects problems in an infant's gut.*[50]99

Wiessinger goes on to make some pretty offensive statements including comparing not breastfeeding to smoking, and arguing that feeling guilty is a natural state for women. The article is a classic among zealous breastfeeding circles.

In the nearly 20 years since Wiessinger first made her case, the language around formula has indeed changed to one of risk. Mothers are repeatedly warned that if they don't breastfeed there is a higher risk of a litany of illnesses. However, there is never any education about exactly how much greater that risk is – there is no discussion of what's known as relative risk. How much more likely is a formula-fed child to get a cold than a breastfed one? And what does that translate to in terms of number of colds per year? We're not told, partially because the evidence is so mixed, and partially, I suspect, because in stark number terms, the risks then wouldn't seem like that big a deal. In a risk culture, that doesn't matter though. Mothers are expected to minimise any risk to their child, no matter how small, or at what cost to herself.

So, when mothers believe they are exposing their child to (exaggerated) risks through formula-feeding, of course guilt is the resulting emotion. Guilt is sometimes even the intended emotion – either to try to bully her into 'trying harder' to breastfeed, or as punishment for the woman who has 'failed' to 'try hard enough' to follow the tenets of intensive motherhood and submit herself entirely to her child's putative well-being, no matter what the cost to herself. In *Bottled Up*, Suzanne Barston dug up a 2005 textbook used for training lactation consultants. The textbook authors discuss the concept of formula-feeding guilt.

> **"**Appropriate guilt can be a positive emotion within the realm of personal growth . . . When you are open and honest with parents regarding the risks of artificial feeding, you will usually find that they appreciate learning what to watch for if they later introduce formula into their baby's diet. You can help parents make guilt work for them as a catalyst to become the best parents they can be.[51] **"**

The admission that lactation consultants feel that guilt is an 'appropriate' emotion to use when trying to encourage mothers to breastfeed, to 'become the best parents they can be', is shocking but not shocking at the same time. This handbook simply codifies the technique of pushing guilt that so many of us have felt from overzealous midwives, doctors, lactation consultants, friends and breastfeeding groups. Of course, if breastfeeding advocates were hoping to improve breastfeeding rates through positioning formula-feeding as risky, they have failed. Since 1996, when Diane Wiessinger's essay came out, rates have increased only slightly. If the real agenda was making formula-feeding parents feel like shit, they've done a bang-up job.

The moralised nature of feeding

There is, however, a popular habit among zealous lactivists to dismiss women feeling guilty about bottle-feeding, with comments along the lines of 'no one can make you feel guilty without your consent', the implication being that lactivists, midwives and health professionals don't *make* women feel guilty, we allow ourselves to feel guilty because we know we have 'committed wrong or failed in an obligation'.[52]

This insidious assertion denies the demonstrable fact that *everything* in our contemporary culture tells us that good mothers breastfeed and bad mothers bottle-feed. Feeding is no longer a practical question, it is a moral one.[53] And as the lactation consultant's handbook shows, the moral authority is not held by a *mother* who decides whether to feel guilty or not, it can be doled out by a quasi-medical professional who tells us what emotions are 'appropriate' for us to feel. Between the misrepresented science, the intensive motherhood ideology that lauds breastfeeding and condemns bottle-feeding, and the risk culture that feeds on the misrepresented science to present bottle-feeding as risky and breastfeeding as safe, what woman with ears, eyes, a brain and a heart could fail to absorb all of this? And when she does, there is only one conclusion – that *not* breastfeeding makes her a bad mother who has failed her child. And who wouldn't feel guilty about that?

Sasha says:

This pressure to breastfeed, and the guilt if you do not, is everywhere for a new mum. From the sad sigh you get from the GP's nurse vaccinating your infant if you say no when she asks you if you are breastfeeding, to your mother-in-law's puzzled look of disappointment as you pull out the bottle of formula, to the kind but slightly patronising pep talk from the health visitor at the baby clinic when you 'confess' you might stop breastfeeding soon, the stigma attached to formula-feeding is inescapable. Unfortunately, the support you need – to breastfeed or to formula-feed – is much harder to come by.

So prevalent is this guilt, sociologists note that not only is it now 'normal' and 'natural', it also serves a purpose. It's a way for formula-feeding mums to show that they are still 'good mothers' because they accept that good mothers breastfeed, and they regret their failure.[54] It has become a coping mechanism. But what a horrible, negative way to cope! I have read stories of mothers who have felt guilty for 30 years because they couldn't and didn't breastfeed. This is so, so wrong.

'I feel really sad about the lack of support and the judgement'

I always intended to breastfeed my daughter. I daydreamed of having my baby snuggled up to my breast in a rocking chair, but as so often happens in life, my dreams weren't realised. I never knew how difficult breastfeeding would be. In fact, I ended up only breastfeeding her for three days, because I had developed pre-eclampsia and high blood pressure. By day four Sophia was mixed-fed bottled breast milk and formula and that's where the guilt started. Even the nurse used to raise an eyebrow at me when I was readmitted to hospital. She asked me if the baby would be brought in to feed and I told her she was at home being formula-fed by her dad. Due to my illness I could only express my milk for three weeks; ever since then she's been formula-fed.

I grieved that I couldn't feed my daughter and I started to lose my initial 'cushy' feelings for my baby. I thought this was because I wasn't breastfeeding and that meant I wasn't properly bonding with my baby. By week seven I was experiencing anxiety attacks that were later diagnosed as postnatal depression. I felt like a failure as a mother for not being able to breastfeed; seeing mothers everywhere breastfeeding made me feel like there was something inherently wrong with me and that I was robbing my baby of something mother nature intended – a sacred bond I would never have with her.

I feel really sad about the lack of support and the judgement. The breastfeeding helpline would not even tell me how to wean off expressing when I told them I was unwell and needed to stop expressing my milk.

I always felt judged by those around me for not breastfeeding, and worst of all by the women at mothers' group! This was so hurtful – as fellow mothers we should support each other, not judge and isolate one another! Their nasty comments about formula-feeding used to see me break down in tears. Even strangers would come up to me in changing rooms and ask if Sophia was breastfed and when I explained she was formula-fed they used to look at me as if I was feeding my baby rat poison.

Now I am fine with it. Guilt is a useless emotion as it changes nothing. We are our own worst critics.

Lori, Sydney, Australia, mother to Sophia, 7 months

Breaking the chains of guilt

It's time to stand up for ourselves. The truth is not only that you shouldn't *feel* guilty for using formula, you are *not* guilty. You have not committed any parenting crime; you are a good mother who loves her baby and is nourishing her.

Formula is not the same as breast milk, but it has been developed over 150 years to allow babies to grow and to develop healthily. Formula-fed babies in the developed world *might* miss out on a few IQ points, *maybe* their ears, noses and tummies are slightly more prone to infection, but formula will not make your baby fat, sick or dumb. Its 'risks' have been vastly overstated, and preyed upon in a risk culture that sets mothers the impossible task of eliminating all possible dangers, no matter how small. The problem is that, as mums, we can never win – everything in life has risks.

There are risks to simply taking your baby outside your front gate – 33 children under 15 died and more than 7,700 were injured as pedestrians in road accidents in the UK in 2011,[55] yet we are not counselled to keep our children inside for their safety. In the United States, over 17,000 children are injured every year by televisions dropping on top of them, yet there is no call to ban TVs.[56]

Breathing polluted city air is 'clearly more toxic than infant formula', writes Jules Law in his analysis 'The politics of breastfeeding', 'but families rarely uproot their lives for incremental reductions in an infant's exposure to carbon monoxide, sulfur dioxide, or lead, and paediatricians are more likely to recommend a practice that will disrupt a woman's career [i.e. breastfeeding] than a relocation that may affect a man's commute.'[57] The 'risks' of bottle-feeding have been given outsized importance, for a number of reasons that have little to do with formula-fed babies' outcomes, and more to do with how we view motherhood, morals and 'natural' versus manufactured products.

So what does this mean for you as you struggle with guilt?

For a start, try to put these 'risks' in perspective. If you are sleeping no more than two hours at a stretch for months on end, is the risk of having your partner give a bottle of formula so you can sleep for four hours straight greater than the risk to your mental state (and therefore potentially your baby's mental state) because of exhaustion? If you are struggling to produce enough milk, what is the greater risk – dehydration or even hypernatraemia of your baby, or the possibility of her dropping a few IQ points because of formula use? (Hypernatraemia is a serious condition caused by a dehydration-related electrolyte imbalance. If untreated, it can lead to seizures, brain damage and death. Breastfeeding-related hypernatraemia, caused by babies not getting enough breast milk, is rare but some researchers worry that it is being missed as a diagnosis.[58])

Sasha says:

As a hospital paediatrician I see babies with hypernatraemia often enough. In its severe form it occurs in less than 1% of newborns, but its frequency appears to have been on the rise over the last 20 years. It usually happens in the first week of life with a first-time mum, exclusively breastfeeding but with not enough milk and a resulting prune-dry, sleepy and potentially unwell infant who needs hospital admission and rehydration with fluids through a drip. The parents are often shocked that their seemingly 'content' baby who has slept most of the first few days of its life is unwell and needs to be in hospital, sometimes for several days. And, of course, it is very hard for a breastfeeding mum to be told that her lack of breast milk has potentially put her infant's life at risk, and these mums usually need a lot of help to regain confidence with breastfeeding once the baby is well again.

We each have to do our own risk analyses according to our own situations, but remember, describing formula as 'risky' has been a deliberate strategy to try to scare women into breastfeeding. Formula is not risky. In the developed world, for full-term babies, its use brings a moderately higher risk of some outcomes. 'Risky' and 'carrying a risk of' are not the same thing. Giving formula is not giving your baby razor blades to juggle.

As parents, we make many choices every day for our children, and because all of them are made within a complex series of interconnecting influences, we can't *always* make the perfect choice *all* the time. We need to give ourselves a break. This is something that Lenore Skenazy reminded me of when I asked her what we should say to worried formula-feeding parents. 'I would say, don't sweat it. You've probably made a million parenting decisions which are fantastic, but nothing can be "optimal". If we had to be raised optimally nobody would be alive because we are human. Most kids turn out okay, and if they don't, it's got nothing to do with whether you breastfed them or not.' It sounds like pretty sensible advice to me.

What about mum? Rebalancing the infant feeding relationship in an era of intensive mothering

As well as re-evaluating the 'risks' of formula, to help kick that guilt to the kerb we need to critically examine the current child-centred, intensive mothering mentality of Western middle-class society, and how that has affected how we feed our babies.

The dogma of intensive motherhood that tells us that women must always put their children's needs before their own dictates that women should do whatever it takes in order to breastfeed their babies. Put aside your need for sleep and body autonomy, forget that mastitis or persistent latching-on pain, ignore the fact that you haven't had time for a shower in three days, don't worry that pumping at work is affecting your job – your baby *needs* that breast milk, and all of your needs are secondary. Perversely, according to this world view, it's almost as though the harder you have to work to breastfeed, the better mother you are. (By the way, this also relates to other aspects of mothering, such as how much pain we are expected to endure during birth. It's not an original comment, but no one advocates painful (rather than pain-*free*) dentistry, do they? Giving birth, one of the few things women do that men can't, is seen as somehow better and purer if it's painful. If men were pushing babies out of their sexual organs, there is no way they would be expected to do it without epidurals.)

There are many things that are wrong with this approach. Firstly, as we've discussed already, it assumes that breast milk is *so* much better than formula that not giving it is negligent. This, as we now know, is untrue. Secondly, it ignores the fact that a mother's needs and her child's needs are inextricably interlinked. A child needs a mother who is healthy, not exhausted, who is happy and stimulated. There is emerging research that indicates that mothers who practise intensive parenting have worse mental health than more laid-back parents[59] – poor maternal mental health can in itself be damaging to babies, defeating the purpose of intensive mothering in the first place.

Even ardent lactivists will agree that if a mother is finding breastfeeding physically and mentally overwhelming, introducing bottles is an acceptable option. The $64,000 question then becomes what is overwhelming? And that, of course, is unanswerable, because no one has ever known what it's like to have *your breasts* and *your baby* and *your story*. But in our culture of intensive mothering, a baby's needs are valued much, much more than a mother's, so the threshold for what is overwhelming or damaging is often unreasonably high.

Sasha says:

And God forbid if you should 'admit' relief at the point when you switched from breastfeeding to formula. The reality is that this is how many women feel on stopping breastfeeding, but revealing this seems to be taken as a sign that you really are a selfish mother. Well, I found it a huge relief and I don't mind admitting it.

So here's a provocative idea – what if, every once in a while, it's okay for a mother to put her needs on an equal footing with those of her child? Or even first? It sounds heretical, but there is actually no law saying kids' needs trump parents' needs every time. We have all been signed up to the intensive motherhood ideology without being asked, simply by being born at a time when it is the prevailing orthodoxy. Going

'I had so much milk, but I used formula so I could go to work'

CASE STUDY

This story comes from my friend Marianne. It's a little different from other stories – she had no troubles breastfeeding, and mixed-fed for a long time – but I like it because she placed value on her own feelings and needs as well as on her children's. And I can safely report she has two divine, smart and very cheeky children who have not suffered in any way because their mum knew that, in order to be a good mother, she needed to fulfil her own needs too.

Beatrix was a delightful surprise – conceived in my final year at uni. However, I was desperate to put my new qualifications to use as well as be a mum. I applied for a job on my due date, and 10 days later, on the same day I gave birth, I found out I had an interview. Imagine the conflicted feelings when, two weeks later, I did the interview and got the job! I was elated and then suddenly shit-scared at the idea of leaving my baby.

I had been a champion breastfeeder, but fortunately Bea also took a bottle and at six weeks I dropped her off at the childminder, happy to take formula or expressed breast milk. She was mixed-fed after that, so that I could go to work. As for the guilt, well, I didn't let myself feel guilty. I wanted, no, needed to work, and if that meant that Bea had to have a bottle, so be it.

Cedric, my deliciously bouncy ginger baby boy, was a whole other kettle of fish. Again, I had no problems breastfeeding. My midwife even brought her colleague in to stare in amazement when I hand-expressed half a cup of colostrum on the first day! But, unlike his sister, Ced refused to take a bottle.

By that stage, we had moved countries and I was a lady of leisure. There was no reason for me to give him a bottle, except that after three months I felt that I needed a day off. After a lot of crying (him and me), and me giving in to his demands for the boob, my husband and I

continued

> *continued from previous page*
>
> hatched a plan where I would go out for the day. I returned that night to find my mother-in-law, a little smugly, giving him a bottle. Initially I felt guilty, but I knew that to be a good mum I needed time off from my kids to recharge and just be me, and if that meant him having a bottle, then again, so be it. He managed to go between bottle and boob pretty easily and I guess I was lucky that I kept my milk supply as I fed him until he was one.
>
> Even though I had so much milk I tried to donate it, I still think that formula is one of the most liberating inventions of all time for women. To any woman struggling with formula guilt, I would say, is your baby safe and loved? If so, don't feel guilty. It's only milk.
>
> Marianne, Kent, mother to Beatrix, 6, and Cedric, 2

against that is hard, it takes guts, but it can be done. It won't make you a bad mother if, every once in a while, you prioritise your own needs. It may in fact make you a better mother.

A good way to start is by listening to the people who love you – your mother, your partner, your friends. As outsiders who aren't down the deep, dark rabbit hole that a new baby can throw us into, they are sometimes in a better position to see what is better for you *as a family*. One of the saddest side effects of the breastfeeding push of the last 50 years is that we are encouraged not to trust our mothers when it comes to caring for our new babies, and especially when it comes to feeding.[60] Our mothers are portrayed as ignorant of the facts, and too ready to suggest formula because that's what they used. One breastfeeding website lists grandmothers as its number one 'booby trap'.[61]

It's true that many of our mothers grew up in an era when breastfeeding was less common, and many of them are less likely to be able to help with the practical aspects, but that doesn't make them stupid. They, too, have read all the stories about how breast milk is so much better than formula. My own mother says she was put under huge pressure to breastfeed when she gave birth to me more than 30 years ago. What they can do, which we sometimes can't, is see the bigger picture. Our mothers, friends and partners want us to achieve our goals because they know that will make us happy, but they might be able to see better whether those goals are realistic. Our loved ones hold our best interests at heart, just like you hold your baby's best interests at heart, so don't be too quick to dismiss them if they tell you they are worried about you.

When I asked Dr Katie Hinde, the researcher who runs Harvard's Comparative Lactation Laboratory, why she thinks so many people are so hostile to formula, she didn't put it down to its risks, as you might expect: she put it down to our intensive mothering culture.

> ❝I think it's because we have a very infant-oriented perspective – that what's best for the infant is of primary importance and greatest value. The woman's role in that is deprived of agency and is basically expected to do whatever is in that infant's best interest, and I think that's a false perspective. Because I think it's important to see breastfeeding choices within a broader matrix of career and society and infrastructure and institutional support. Yes, breastfeeding is almost always going to be the healthiest physiological feeding choice for that baby, but that's not the only thing that needs to be considered in that dynamic.[62]❞

It's a refreshing antidote to the view of breastfeeding zealots that 'breastfeeding is superior to artificial feeding in all places, at all times, and for all women'.[63]

It's time to bring a little more balance to the relationship between mothers and babies, especially when it comes to feeding. The only way we are going to stem the epidemic of guilt among formula-feeding mothers is by tempering the view that in order to be good parents we must sacrifice everything of ourselves, for the higher purpose of our child. That's the same attitude found in religious fundamentalists who do crazy, dangerous things in the name of their god. Babies are not gods. They are beautiful, vulnerable little human beings who need us to love them, feed them and nurture them. As long as we are doing all of those things, then we have no reason to *feel* guilty, because we are *not* guilty.

Conclusion

The view in our toddler-shaped rear-view mirrors

6 November 2013. I am hunched over a computer, searching on parenting forums for answers, asking friends for advice. I'm spending hours looking at my child, evaluating her. I'm reporting triumphs and failures on Facebook, receiving sympathy, pats on the back, encouragement to keep going and assurances that there's no harm in stopping. No, I am not breastfeeding or bottle-feeding my daughter. I'm toilet training her.

Two years after my beautiful baby was born, the questions and the anxieties about whether I am doing the right thing haven't gone away, they have just taken a different focus. Now, instead of worrying about whether I am pumping enough to stimulate my flow, or whether I should be using an organic formula, I'm dealing with how to get her to eat broccoli, worrying about her still refusing to share her toys with her cousins and fretting about whether her nursery stimulates her enough.

It may seem impossible to believe if you're still in the new baby bubble, but one day you won't spend your entire day thinking and worrying about feeding. One day, you'll wake up and realise that you and your baby have made it through those first few months, and whether you're using breast or bottle, you've both got the hang of this feeding thing. Instead, you'll realise you're starting to think about different things – weaning, crawling, childcare and first words.

I still laugh when I remember a conversation with my lovely lawyer neighbour, Camilla, when my daughter was one week old. Camilla was playing with her little 18-month-old in our communal garden, and she came up and asked how I was doing. 'So happy, but pretty tired,'

I replied in a slightly desperate tone. Our daughter had kept us up every night that week between midnight and 5 a.m., as she cried with hunger because I was stupidly still trying to exclusively breastfeed her. Camilla looked at me in her wonderfully deadpan way. 'Look, what you must realise is that these are the worst six weeks of your life,' she said. 'I mean, of course they're wonderful, and you have to say they're wonderful, but actually they are the worst. You're just so tired, and you have no idea what you're doing. It's awful.'

I laughed, but I must have looked a little bit scared too, because she then added, 'But it gets better. So much better. You just have to get through these six weeks.'

And do you know what? She was right. I had six weeks of increasing desperation and exasperation. There were days when I felt I didn't get off the couch because I was spending so much time feeding, topping up, expressing, just in time to start the whole cycle again. And in those moments when I did make it off the couch, it was only to go to the laundry to put on another load of vomit-stained clothes. But then, six weeks in, just as I thought I couldn't take it anymore, my baby smiled at me. Not a milk-drunk smile, or a falling-asleep smile, a proper 'pleased-to-meet-you' smile. That made the sleep deprivation worthwhile. Not long after, I made the decision that I was going to spend more time enjoying my baby, and less time on a futile quest for breast milk that was simply never going to succeed. It was the right decision. Because as I have watched my predominantly formula-fed baby grow into a happy, healthy toddler, and seen her friends who were all fed in different ways grow up too, I can honestly say that in the big scheme of things, it really doesn't matter.

Throughout this book we have acknowledged that evidence shows that there are differences between bottle-fed and breastfed babies, with breastfed babies being, in the main, moderately healthier. But we have also shown you that for those of us lucky enough to live in the developed world, the benefits of breastfeeding have been exaggerated.

Formula allowed my baby to thrive when I couldn't physically give her the breast milk she needed. Perhaps in your case formula will have been what allowed you to go back to work to support your baby, or what stopped you from going crazy with exhaustion or feeding pain, or what helped you continue to breastfeed, or simply what enabled you to feel like you were in control of your own body again. These are not reasons to feel guilty; they are reasons to feel grateful that we live in a time when bottle-feeding is a safe, readily available, nutritionally complete option.

Our aim throughout this book has been not to simply pat you on the head and tell you that you *shouldn't feel guilty*, as other books will, but to show you why *you are not guilty*. As a society, we have got ourselves into this crazy position where how we feed our babies has come to define whether we see ourselves as good mothers or not. We hope that we have also shown you why this is so, so wrong.

I have had researchers and academics decline to be interviewed for this book, even as they tell me it is a very worthwhile and much needed project. In giving their apologies, they say they're worried that being quoted in a work that tells women it's okay to feed their babies formula could damage their reputations, or be misinterpreted as not supporting breastfeeding. It is truly a sad indictment on our society that in order to promote breastfeeding, we think we can't even acknowledge the value and the safety of the alternative.

It's time to grow up. We must continue to fight to normalise breast-feeding and to protect it. That means better support of breast feeding mothers, not just in hospital, but throughout society: more midwives and health visitors, so they can have the time to give the help they want to; free, ongoing lactation consultants and better maternity provisions at work; giving an encouraging smile to the woman nervously unclipping her nursing bra in a cafe; and if you are breastfeeding yourself, doing it in front of other people to help normalise it. It also means continuing to work to stop formula companies preying on vulnerable mothers, in both the developed and the developing worlds. But it also means providing more realistic education about what breastfeeding is really like, and letting it be simply something mothers enjoy doing, rather than something they must do, because of exaggerated benefits.

We also need to acknowledge that in our modern world many of us use formula, not because we are lazy, or have fallen for marketing tricks, but because it is the best option for our family within the complex matrix of interweaving influences that govern our daily life. We need better, more easily accessible information about how to choose a formula, safely prepare it, and give a bottle with love. We need personalised, realistic feeding plans, which take into account the many variables of our pregnancies, births, families and work circumstances. We need to rebalance the intensive mothering dogma that says women must always put their own needs last, and they must do whatever it takes to minimise any risk, no matter how small, and portrays breastfeeding as always good and formula-feeding as always bad. And above all, we need, and indeed deserve, not to be judged for our choices. That also means not judging ourselves.

Whether you are breastfeeding at 2 years, mixed-feeding at four months, or formula-feeding at day one, if you know that you are doing what is right for your family, then that is all that matters. Only you and your partner can judge what is best for your own circumstances.

And remember: feeding does not determine your baby's future – the biggest influence over your child's life is what sort of parent you choose to be. The best start for your baby doesn't come from a breast or a bottle, it comes from your heart. As long as you put all of *that* into raising your child, that's all that truly matters.

Sasha says:

When Madeleine first asked me to be a part of *Guilt-free Bottle-feeding*, I was intrigued, enthused and excited. The inspiration for the book had emerged in large part from Madeleine's own personal story, and I had many shared and personal experiences that I wanted to add to that story. But the book you have here is neither about us nor for us; it has grown into something much more. I have talked about the 'message' of GFBF time and time again over the course of it being written: with family, friends, colleagues, academics and even patients. And each and every time the response has been that such a book is really *needed*; that they or their wife or sister or best friend would have really benefited from such a book because that woman had also had a difficult feeding story with her own child. It makes me so sad to hear of so many women whose first few months with their baby have been harder, sadder and more painful than they needed to be. Tough times that could have been eased if only they had been properly informed prenatally about what feeding methods might be right for them; if only they had been properly supported to feed in the way they wanted to and not pressured to do what wasn't right for them and their baby. With the knowledge about what the true differences are between breastfeeding and bottle-feeding, and with the shared experiences and support that this book provides, I hope we can take a few steps towards more mums being better informed and having the confidence to find your own personal 'right' way through those first few months of the hardest and most amazing thing you'll ever have the privilege to do, to be a mum.

Part 2

The practice

1 Choosing a formula

Formula-feeding or mixed feeding can be nerve-wracking because there is so little unbiased, freely accessible information. We have written this second part of *Guilt-free Bottle-feeding* to try to bridge some of this gap.[1]

We have collated the best information available from the most reliable sources to give you a safe starting point on your feeding journey, but you will likely have questions that aren't answered here. Your trusted health professional should be your first point of contact for all questions relating to the health of your baby, including feeding.

> ### First Steps Nutrition Trust
>
> Because of the large number of formulas and their ever changing ingredients, it's not possible to list them all here. However, the First Steps Nutrition Trust is an excellent source of frequently updated, unbiased information on formulas and feeding and we recommend you consult their website before choosing a formula: firststepsnutrition.org. Joining online or face-to-face support groups such as BottleBabies.org is also a great way to receive support, learn what works for other parents and share your own experiences. Please consult the Resources section of this book on page 201 for a list of reliable organisations and websites that can provide more information on specific topics.

Formula basics

- Every commercially available formula contains a combination of proteins, fat, carbohydrates and vitamins and minerals. Some have added optional extras such as pre- and probiotics, long-chain polyunsaturated fatty acids and nucleotides.

- Formulas are regulated by national governments or health authorities, which generally prescribe minimum and maximum amounts of energy values, proteins, fats, vitamins and minerals, and say what ingredients can be used. They also say which optional extras can be added. However, in the UK it is possible for formula companies to add extras prior to receiving approval from health authorities.

- Formulas can come in powdered form, in concentrate (rare these days) and in ready-to-feed cartons of liquid. Each form has its own advantages and disadvantages (see page 170).

- Pre-made ready-to-feed formula is sterile; powdered formula is not. Powdered formula needs to be prepared in a way that kills off any potential bacteria.

- The World Health Organization (WHO) recommends that ready-to-feed liquid formula be given to all babies under two months rather than powdered formula, because of the risk of bacterial contamination of powdered formula.[2]

- Most infant formulas are made out of modified cow's milk. Some are made out of soya milk and a few out of goat's milk. There are a number of specialist milks where the milk is processed in a different way; these can be given to babies who have difficulty taking regular formula after consultation with a health professional.

- Because the content of formula is heavily regulated, there are only marginal differences between different formulas, mostly in the optional extras they contain. However, you will probably find that your baby digests some better than others.

- There is no formula that is 'closest to breast milk'. Formula is modelled on breast milk, but due to breast milk's live nature and extensive number of ingredients, it cannot be replicated.

- The ingredients for formula can come from many different sources and can change between batches. Companies are not required to state the origin of their ingredients or when it changes.

Regular cow's milk infant formulas for babies under six months (stage 1)

What's in infant formula?

Protein

- **Whey** and **casein** are the two main proteins in both breast milk and infant formulas. Whey empties faster from the stomach because it remains in liquid form, which means that it is easier to digest. Casein curdles in the stomach, which means it requires more work and takes longer to digest.
- In colostrum and early breast milk, whey is dominant – the ratio is 60% whey and 40% casein. Cow's milk is naturally casein-dominant, with 20% whey and 80% casein. When making stage 1 milks, formula manufacturers change the whey to casein ratio of cow's milk to make it the same as that of breast milk. This is one big difference between formula and regular cow's milk.

Baby struggling with stage 1 formula?

If your baby is having trouble digesting regular infant formula (she has wind or is more constipated than normal), look at the whey to casein ratio. Moving to one with a whey content above the standard 60% of standard stage 1 milks might be one way to improve the situation.

- Contained within proteins are **amino acids**, which help our bodies to develop. Breast milk has higher concentrations of some essential amino acids that cannot be produced by the body and therefore need to be ingested.
- In order to get the necessary amounts of these amino acids, formula has traditionally had a higher concentration of protein than breast milk does. While this helps to make sure babies are getting the amino acids they need, it has the downside of promoting faster growth in babies, which can make children more likely to become overweight. To try to counter this problem, most formulas now contain proteins at the lower end of the scale allowed by the European Union (EU), and some are adding α-lactalbumin (see below).

Fats

- Fats make up 50% of the energy source of formula, which is about the same as mature human milk. The fats in formula typically come from vegetable oils, although fish and fungus oils are also used.
- The fats found in cow's milk and breast milk are very different, so cow's milk is manipulated to reduce some elements, and other elements are added in the formula production process to get it closer to the fat profile of breast milk.
- Breast milk is higher in unsaturated fats, and has long-chain polyunsaturated fatty acids (LCPUFAs), arachidonic acid (ARA), eicosapentaenoic acid and docosahexaenoic acid (DHA). These fats help eye and brain development. Non-organic infant baby formulas often have added LCPUFAs, although there is mixed evidence on whether they are worth the extra money. (See page 63 for more on this.)

Carbohydrates

- **Lactose** is the main carbohydrate of both breast milk and formula and provides about 40% of the energy. Some formulas have added lactose if they have been made from skimmed milk powder. Lactose is helpful to digestion, although a few babies have a lactose intolerance.
- **Glucose** is used as a carbohydrate in formulas for babies with a lactose intolerance, although it is generally not suitable for babies.
- **Maltodextrin** is another carbohydrate source frequently found in formulas. It mostly comes from corn or potatoes and is easily digestible.

Vitamins and minerals

- Vitamins and minerals are essential for healthy growth. Because most can't be produced by the body, they need to be ingested through food.
- The vitamins and minerals found in all infant formulas must be in minimum and maximum quantities set by health authorities.
- Some vitamins and minerals found in breast milk, such as **calcium** and **zinc**, are more easily absorbed than when they are found in formula, so higher levels are added.
- Some vitamins and minerals deteriorate during storage, so make sure you always follow the 'use by' date on the tin. Formulas have additives to reduce the deterioration of vitamins and minerals.

- **Iron** was previously believed to be absorbed more poorly from formula than from breast milk, so stage 1 infant formula has traditionally had nearly 10 times the iron levels of breast milk. However, new evidence suggests that it is actually absorbed at the same rate, regardless of whether it comes from breast milk or formula, so there is now some concern about the higher level of iron in infant milks because iron can stop other minerals being absorbed properly and is one of the causes of constipation in formula-fed babies.

- Follow-on formulas have even higher levels of iron, and this is one of the reasons why the UK government recommends that babies stay on stage 1 infant formula until they are a year old, rather than changing to follow-on formula. This is also because many other foods babies receive from the age of six months will be fortified with iron, so there is the potential for very high iron intake, which can be harmful to development.

Additives

- Most formulas contain additives that are needed to make sure that powders don't separate, that acidity is regulated, and that ingredients resist oxidation. Other additives thicken formula and stop casein coagulating. These additives are approved by the EU for adult use; however, not all of them have been tested for use on children.

Optional extras that may be found in stage 1 formula milks

Nucleotides are added to all non-organic stage 1 formula milks in the UK. They are involved in regulating metabolism and energy transfer and are the building blocks of DNA. Different formulas have different percentages of nucleotides added to them. Your body naturally produces some, but at times of rapid growth, such as in infancy, it may not be able to make as many as are needed, so they need to be supplemented. Breast milk has more nucleotides than cow's milk and they are different in structure. It is believed that nucleotides play a role in both the immune and gastrointestinal systems, and some studies report that babies fed nucleotide-supplemented formulas have fewer tummy troubles and respond better to some vaccinations. However, the evidence for this is not yet clear-cut.

Galacto-oligosaccharides (GOS) and **fructo-oligosaccharides (FOS)** are **prebiotics** that can be added to formula with the aim of improving gut health. Breast milk is rich in prebiotic oligosaccharides that promote the growth and activity of healthy bacteria in the gut, which in turn affect the overall health of the baby. Regular cow's milk formula contains virtually none. The synthetically produced GOS and FOS that are added to some formulas are not the same as breast milk oligosaccharides, but their addition has been shown to promote healthy gut bacteria at the expense of some harmful gut bacteria. It's good to choose a formula with prebiotics if you can.

Long-chain polyunsaturated fatty acids are sometimes written as **LCPUFAs** or **DHA** (docosahexaenoic acid), **ARA** (arachidonic acid) or **Omega-3** and **Omega-6**. LCPUFAs promote healthy brain and eye growth, although there is some debate about whether the particular types added to formula milk have a benefit. There is no evidence that they do harm. See page 63 for a further discussion of this.

'Gold' formulas

'Gold' formula is the name sometimes given to formula with the added optional extras above. It's a name commonly used in Australia to differentiate these formulas from standard ones.

α-lactalbumin is a whey protein that contains essential amino acids and is added to some formulas. Formulas with α-lactalbumin have a lower protein content than standard formulas, which could reduce some of the risk of rapid weight gain among formula-fed babies. It's likely that more formula companies will add α-lactalbumin in the future to allow them to have a lower protein count. However, at the time of writing, there has not been enough research into the effect of adding α-lactalbumin to conclusively say that it has benefits.

Betapol is added to some formulas. It is a structured vegetable oil that is promoted as aiding constipation and improving calcium absorption. There are a number of studies that indicate it does this, although other studies show no difference. Not all formulas that contain Betapol market it as such, so even if your formula doesn't say it is added on the tin, it may still contain the substance. It might refer to it as a 'special vegetable fat blend', a 'new fat blend' or 'SN-2 enriched fat blend'.

Probiotics are live micro-organisms that also help to promote gut health. At the time of writing, no stage 1 formula milks in the UK add probiotics. This is because probiotic-supplemented formula needs to be made up with water heated to a maximum of 50° Celsius in order to keep the probiotic active, and this contravenes the Department of Health's recommendation that all formula be made up with water that is boiled and then left to cool to no less than 70° Celsius to kill off potential contaminants.

Taurine is a free amino acid (a building block of protein) that is added to most infant milks, although it is not compulsory. It is found in abundance in breast milk, but not in cow's milk. Even though there has been no clear clinical benefit demonstrated for it, taurine has been added to formula for decades because its addition allowed companies to patent their formulas. There doesn't appear to be any harm from supplemented taurine.

Lutein is an antioxidant that can help protect the eye. At the moment, it is not allowed in formulas in the UK, although it is in Australia and could potentially be added to formulas in the future.

Organic formulas

The main difference with organic formulas is that they are made out of organic milk, which is free of pesticides and produced in a more sustainable fashion. Some organic formulas don't add certain optional extras such as DHA and ARA because of concerns over the way they are produced. There is no solid evidence that organic formulas are significantly better for babies than regular formulas. Organic formulas cost more.

Impressive branding? Check the ingredients

Formula companies sometimes make up fancy names for the extra ingredients they put into their milks. The aim of this is to make a more impressive-sounding product, which you will then be more likely to choose. Often, the name will be trademarked, and the product may well cost more. However, before you snap it up, check what this impressive ingredient actually consists of. It may well just be a name given to the particular mix of ingredients they use, such as GOS and LCPUFAs, and that may well be found in other formula brands too, though just without the trademarked name. This is all completely legal, but you need to be aware that this is a common marketing tool.

Other formulas suitable from birth

Hungry baby formula

Most formula companies also make hungry baby formula for infants who seem to always want to feed. If your baby is feeding very frequently and gaining too much weight, you can try a hungry baby formula; however, it's a good idea to talk to your health professional first.

The dominant protein in hungry baby formulas is casein (rather than whey, which is dominant in regular stage 1 milks and breast milk). Because casein takes longer to work its way through the gut, the theory is that it keeps a baby fuller for longer. However, the evidence supporting this claim is not very strong.

Hungry baby formulas have slightly higher carbohydrate and protein ratios, balanced by slightly lower fat ratios, to give them about the same energy values as regular formula. The vitamins and mineral ratios are also slightly different; however, all hungry baby formulas fall within the guidelines for nutritional profile.

Very young babies might find hungry baby formula too hard to digest because of the higher casein content, and even older babies might have the same problem. This could lead to them being unsettled and uncomfortable. If you're worried about your baby's feeding, the best thing to do is speak to a health professional before chopping and changing formulas too regularly.

Anti-reflux formula

Reflux describes when babies repeatedly bring up feed into their oesophagus, or repeatedly spit up or vomit more than normal.

Anti-reflux formulas are regular formulas that have been thickened by adding rice, corn starch or carob bean gum. The whey to casein ratio of anti-reflux formulas is 20:80.

In the UK, anti-reflux formulas are available on prescription or can be bought over the counter at a pharmacy without prescription.

Anti-reflux formulas will tend to go lumpy if made up with water that is 70° Celsius, so manufacturers recommend that it is made up at a lower temperature. As a parent, you need to weigh up the risks of potential bacterial infection from formula made up at a lower temperature against the potential benefits of reduced reflux.

While some studies show that thickened baby formula can help with reflux, the European Society of Paediatric Gastroenterology, Hepatology and Nutrition doesn't recommend its use.

Should I use anti-reflux formula?

Bringing up small amounts of milk after a feed is normal. If you are concerned about your baby's vomiting or spitting up, your first port of call should be a health professional, rather than simply buying an anti-reflux formula. Reflux can be distressing for both baby and parents, and it is best discussed with a doctor or nurse, who will be able to suggest ways of feeding and coping with reflux that don't necessarily involve changing formulas.

Lactose-free formula

The main carbohydrate in formula is lactose, but a very small number of babies are lactose intolerant. Lactose intolerance is caused by an imbalance between the amount of lactose ingested and the ability of the enzyme lactase to process it in the body. Symptoms of lactose intolerance can include tummy pain, diarrhoea, flatulence and bloating. It is more common among black and Asian populations, and may occur for a short time after a gastrointestinal infection.

In lactose-free formulas, the carbohydrate lactose is replaced with glucose. Lactose-free formula is available over the counter from pharmacies.

Lactose-free formulas are nutritionally complete and suitable from birth. However, because glucose is used, there is a much higher risk of dental caries (holes) than from regular formula. Babies on lactose-free formula should avoid prolonged milk feeds and should always have their teeth cleaned after the last feed at night.

If you think your baby may be lactose intolerant, speak to your doctor or nurse before changing formulas.

Partially hydrolysed formula

Partially hydrolysed formulas are based on modified cow's milk and can be based on either whey or casein proteins or a mixture of both. The proteins have been partially broken down into smaller fragments (hydrolysed), making them easier to digest.

They are often referred to as 'comfort' milks or 'easier to digest' and are freely available in supermarkets. In the UK at the time of writing, all partially hydrolysed formulas are 100% whey protein. They are considerably more expensive than regular milks.

Partially hydrolysed formulas are marketed as being suitable for babies with colic or constipation; however, the evidence for these claims is not overly robust. If your baby is experiencing excessive gas or constipation, you can try a partially hydrolysed formula, but make sure you also try the suggestions to relieve these common formula side effects listed on page 197.

Partially hydrolysed formula is sometimes suggested as a solution for reducing the risk of allergies in children with a family history of allergic disease. Some companies market partially hydrolysed formula as helping to reduce the risk of atopic dermatitis; however, Britain's National Institute for Health and Clinical Excellence concluded in 2008 that there is 'insufficient evidence that infant formulas based on partially or extensively hydrolysed cow's milk protein can prevent allergies'.[3] If you have a family history of allergies and are worried about your baby's chances of developing an allergy, speak to a health professional.

Partially hydrolysed formula is not hypoallergenic and *should not be given to babies with a cow's milk allergy*.

Milk protein allergy or lactose intolerance?

An allergy or intolerance to cow's milk protein is different from lactose intolerance. Milk allergy or intolerance is an allergic reaction; lactose intolerance is not – it's an enzyme deficiency and is more uncommon. Milk allergy can be serious and if your baby displays symptoms you should see a doctor. Symptoms include: diarrhoea, nausea and vomiting, eczema and rashes, nasal congestion, wheezing, coughing, loose stools, poor feeding and anaphylaxis.

Extensively hydrolysed formula (protein hydrolysate formula)

The proteins in extensively hydrolysed formula have been broken down even more than in partially hydrolysed formula and are the *first choice for babies who are allergic to cow's milk*. Statistics suggest that between 3% and 8% of infants may have a genuine cow's milk allergy or intolerance.

Hydrolysed formulas are much more expensive than regular formulas but are available on prescription from the NHS.

Breaking down the proteins so much can make the milk taste bitter. Some extensively hydrolysed formulas add fructose to make it taste better, but these are only suitable for babies older than six months. Babies on hydrolysed formulas will have unpleasant poos.

There is some evidence that babies fed hydrolysed protein formulas gain weight at a similar rate to breastfed babies, whereas babies fed regular formula gain weight more rapidly. There is also some evidence that babies with a family history of allergy are less likely to have allergies as children if they received hydrolysed formula rather than regular formula.

Anecdotal evidence from mums suggests that, unfortunately, some GPs don't know much about the differences between specialist formulas and how to treat allergies in infants. If you feel your baby has an allergy and needs a specialist formula, you may need to ask for a referral to a paediatrician.

Hypoallergenic amino-acid formula

These formulas are for babies with extreme allergies to cow's milk and other food protein intolerances. They do not contain any cow's milk protein; instead, they have free amino acids (which are the building blocks of protein) with added nutrients.

These formulas are expensive but are available on prescription on the NHS.

Soya formula

Babies who are lactose intolerant or who have a cow's milk protein allergy are sometimes recommended to go onto a soya formula. Soya formulas are made from soya beans, and the carbohydrate source is glucose rather than lactose.

A significant proportion of babies who are allergic to cow's milk protein will also be allergic to soya protein.

Soya formulas *aren't* recommended for babies under the age of six months, unless prescribed by a medical practitioner. This is because of concerns about potential allergic reactions, the natural presence of phyto-oestrogens, which could potentially affect the hormonal system, and the use of glucose as the energy source.

Talk to a health professional if you are worried that your baby might be allergic to regular formula. In most cases, particularly if your baby is young, a hydrolysed formula is the better option.

Goat's milk formula

Goat's milk formulas were permitted by the EU food regulator in 2012 after previously being found unsuitable for babies. The UK is changing its laws to follow this directive. Goat's milk formulas are available in Australia.

Goat's milk formulas are not lactose-free formulas; they contain similar levels of lactose to cow's milk formulas and are not suitable for babies with a lactose allergy or intolerance.

Goat's milk proteins are different from cow's milk proteins and may or may not be more easily digested by babies with a cow's milk protein allergy – it depends on the baby.

Anecdotally, some families find that goat's milk formula, or a combination of goat's and cow's milk formula, is more easily digested and reduces outbreaks of atopy, such as eczema, but current findings from the European Food Safety Authority (EFSA) say there is not enough evidence to support these claims.

Homemade formulas

It may sound wacky but there are a number of websites that give recipes for homemade formulas, usually using raw (unprocessed) milk, oils and extra vitamins. *It is not recommended that you make these milks.*

Raw animal milks in particular carry a number of bacteria that can be harmful to babies. As much as we may not like the idea of supporting big formula companies, or giving our babies additives, formula regulations are strict and have been compiled after decades of research to give babies a safe, complete form of nutrition. Homemade formulas are unregulated, highly variable in content and untested for appropriate levels of nutrients.

If you are very opposed to using commercially produced formula, then by far your better option is to use donated breast milk for your baby.

Formulas for babies older than six months

Follow-on formula (stage 2) basics

- Follow-on formulas are marketed for babies over the age of six months who have started to be weaned onto solids as well as milk. Their nutritional composition is regulated by governments.
- Formula companies aggressively market follow-on milks. Because they are not allowed to advertise stage 1 milks under the WHO marketing code, they attempt to build brand awareness through other products, including follow-on milks.
- Follow-on milks contain more protein, iron and micronutrients than stage 1 milks. However, as long as babies are eating a diverse,

age-appropriate, complementary diet that contains sufficient iron, protein, fats and nutrients, it is generally agreed that there is no need for babies to move on to follow-on milks. For this reason, *current UK feeding guidelines recommend that babies older than six months continue to receive stage 1 milks rather than follow-on milks until they are 1 year old.*

- Follow-on milks have a high iron content. While babies over the age of six months need more iron than when they were younger, too much iron is bad for babies as it reduces the uptake of other nutrients. In babies who already have enough iron in their diets, using an iron-fortified milk has been shown to impact negatively on cognitive outcomes later in childhood.[4] Babies older than six months can get plenty of iron by drinking stage 1 milks and including green leafy vegetables, meat and legumes in their diet as they are weaned onto solids.

- The UK Department of Health recommends that all children between the ages of six months and five years be given vitamin drops, and this is one way of ensuring that your baby gets all the nutrition she needs, even if she is a fussy eater, without using follow-on formula.

Cow's milk, goat's milk, regular soya milk and nut milks should not be given to babies under the age of one, although they can be used in cooking from six months.

Growing-up milk (stage 3) and toddler milk basics

- Growing-up milks are marketed for children over the age of 1 year. Toddler milks are marketed for children over the age of 2. There are no regulated guidelines on the composition of growing-up and toddler milks.

- These milks are heavily marketed by formula companies; however, *for healthy toddlers and children receiving a normal diet, there is no need for growing-up milks.* Children over a year old can be gradually moved on to full-fat cow's milk in their bottles and cups.

- Growing-up milks contain higher quantities of some nutrients than cow's milk; however, more nutrients doesn't necessarily mean better. Because children over the age of one should be getting most of their nutritional needs from solids, not milk, as long as they have a diverse, normal diet they should receive all the nutrients they need from the combination of cow's milk and food. An excess of some nutrients, such as iron, can actually be harmful.

- Growing-up milks are generally high in sugar and taste much sweeter than cow's milk. This can put children at higher risk of tooth decay. It can also give your children a preference for very sweet drinks.

- If you're worried that your child is a fussy eater and isn't getting enough nutrients, remember that fussiness over food is a very normal stage for toddlers and that they will generally grow out of it. Children, as a general rule, will not let themselves starve. If you are very worried about your child's eating habits, speak to a child health nurse. They will be able to recommend a course of action, which may include a toddler milk.

- For children over the age of one who are unable to take cow's milk, standard unsweetened calcium-fortified soya milk or unsweetened nut-based milks are alternatives, but you should speak to a child health nurse or a paediatric nutritionist first. Rice milks are not recommended for children under five because they can contain high levels of arsenic.

Powdered versus ready-to-feed

Parents can choose either powdered or ready-to-feed liquid formula. Each has advantages and disadvantages, which need to be weighed up. Often, parents use a mixture of the two, preparing powdered formula at home and using ready-to-feeds when out and about.

The WHO recommends using ready-to-feed formula for babies under two months who aren't being breastfed because of the reduced risk of infection. This is a good idea if you can afford it, but needs to be weighed against the considerable extra expense of ready-to-feed formula.

Powdered versus ready-to-feed formula

Powdered	Ready-to-feed
Needs to be reconstituted with water	Already in liquid form and ready to be given to baby
Risk of incorrect reconstitution	No risk of incorrect reconstitution
Not sterile – needs to be prepared with boiled water allowed to cool to 70° Celsius to kill any potential bacteria, including salmonella and *Cronobacter sakazakii*	Sterile until opened, and recommended by WHO for use for babies under 2 months
Greater risk of infection from poor preparation, particularly to newborns with immature immune systems	Less risk of infection, particularly to newborns, because it is sterile until opened
Less convenient due to the time needed to safely make up bottles	More convenient – ready to put into clean, sterilised bottles at any time
Less expensive	Considerably more expensive
Less waste – parents can prepare the exact amount they expect to need	More waste – parents frequently throw away unused formula that cannot be stored for longer than 24 hours in a fridge once opened
Limited shelf life – check the 'use by' date	Must be used within 24 hours once opened and stored in a fridge below 5° Celsius

Bacteria in powdered infant formula

There have been a number of instances of infant formula being found to contain the dangerous bacteria *Cronobacter sakazakii* and salmonella. Cronobacter can cause blood infections, meningitis and necrotising enterocolitis and can be fatal. Salmonella infections can cause diarrhoea and vomiting, which can be severe in babies.

These infections are very rare: in healthy weight babies in the US, the WHO reports that there is 1 case of cronobacter infection for every 100,000 infants, and 140 cases of salmonellosis for every 100,000 infants[5] – not all of these infections are related to formula. *Cronobacter sakazakii* isn't only found in formula tins – it can live elsewhere in the kitchen, in soil and around the house.

Although very rare, infections can have severe consequences, which is why formula guidelines always recommend making up feeds with water boiled and cooled to no less than 70° Celsius to kill off the bacteria. Formula manufacturers make every effort to stop contamination of their formula, but cronobacter in particular has been found to survive for a long time in powdered formula tins.

Other less dangerous bacteria can also live in powdered formula and baby bottles.

How bacteria grow

Bacteria can grow rapidly between the temperatures of 7° Celsius and 65° Celsius, which is why a lukewarm bottle of milk is an ideal breeding ground. This is why all unused formula must be thrown out after two hours (at the latest) and not put back in the fridge. Even if a bottle started off with safe levels of bacteria, after two hours at room temperature the bacteria may have multiplied to a level that could be harmful to your baby. Putting that bottle in the fridge does not kill the bacteria – they remain there, ready to be drunk by your baby if you re-use the bottle. Water boiled and allowed to cool to 70° Celsius kills off pretty much all bacteria, which is why guidelines recommend that water be added to formula powder at this temperature. However, if it is much hotter it can kill off some of the nutrients, so use a sterilised thermometer if necessary to check water temperature.

Changing formulas

If you find that a particular formula isn't suiting your baby (see 'Feeding' on page 185 for signs to look out for) then you should change it. Little tummies often find that an abrupt change can be hard to take, so start by mixing in a small amount of your new formula with your regular one, and gradually change the ratios over a few days so that eventually you're left with just the new one. Doing the maths with different scoop sizes and water volumes can be tricky, so be careful.

It can take a couple of days before you'll know if the new formula is suiting your baby better, especially if you are changing ratios gradually, so don't throw your hands in the air if you don't immediately see an improvement in her poo, wind, constipation or other signs of distress.

If a doctor recommends that you should change formula immediately if your baby has an intolerance or an allergy, then of course you should do that. And if you find that your baby is having constant troubles with formula above and beyond the normal slight constipation and wind, then see a health professional.

2 Choosing a bottle

Once you've decided which formula to use, you are faced with your next big decision – which bottle. Again, the choice is wide, with each brand promising that theirs is the best for fussy babies, colicky babies, mixed-fed babies, the list goes on. In truth, you won't know which one is right for your baby until you try, and I have friends who haven't hit on the right one until bottle brand number five. It can get expensive, so before you buy your full complement of six bottles, matching teats and steriliser, it's worth buying just a couple of one particular brand to try for a few days to see if it works. Many midwives I have spoken to are sceptical about the benefits of more expensive anti-colic bottles, but some mums swear by them. Again, you won't know until you try.

Because the range of bottles is so wide and ever-growing, we can provide you with only a generalised guide here. Baby websites often contain reviews of specific bottles that can be helpful.

Bottle basics

Bottles are made up of three parts: the teat, the collar or ring and the bottle itself. The teat fits into the collar which then screws onto the bottle. You will generally need to buy parts of the same brand so that they fit.

The bottle

- Bottles can be wide- or narrow-necked. Wide-necked ones are generally easier to prepare and wash (something you'll be doing a lot of) while narrow-necked ones are easier for babies to hold once they reach the age when they can hold their own bottles.
- You should always choose bottles that are bisphenol A (BPA)-free. BPA is a chemical used to harden plastics that has been associated

with a higher cancer risk. Most bottles these days are BPA-free but double-check before you buy one – it will say so on the box.

- Most bottles will have a venting system, which allows air to flow back into the bottle to ensure a regular flow of milk, and to prevent babies swallowing too much air when they suck. Some bottles, such as Avent and Nuk, have the vent built into the teat; others, such as Dr Brown's, have a more complicated venting system. Again, which one works for you will be a case of trial and error. Bear in mind that more complicated bottle systems are more difficult to clean.

- It's a good idea to choose a bottle that you can easily get replacements for, as you'll need to replace them after a couple of months as they start to become scratched, especially if you are using plastic ones. Don't use bottles handed down from another sibling or friend.

- Babies need only small feeds when they are born, so if you're using bottles from birth you can buy smaller ones that take a maximum of 100 ml. This is optional.

Glass bottles – a new (old) option

Scientists aren't just worried about the effect of BPA on our health. They are becoming increasingly concerned about the effect of other everyday chemicals, including phthalates, which are commonly used in baby bottles. There are worries that other chemicals found in plastics are affecting our fertility, cancer risk and weight, but there isn't yet enough research to conclude side effects one way or another. What we do know is that the older and more scratched plastic bottles get, the more they leach chemicals, which is why you should always replace bottles after a couple of months or when they start looking scratched.

If you don't like the idea of your baby constantly feeding out of a plastic container, there is an increasing number of glass bottles available that contain no potentially harmful chemicals. Plastic also leaches chemicals when heated, especially in a microwave, but glass doesn't, so glass bottles are a good option if you are worried about reducing your baby's chemical exposure.

The teat

- The makers of wide-necked bottles with flat-ish teats market them as being closer to breasts, but the most important thing is that your baby has a good latch around the nipple that doesn't let in air and allows her to drink comfortably. This could be from either a wide- or a narrow-necked bottle (see below).

- Teats can be made of latex (yellow/brown) or silicone (clear). Latex teats are softer and may be better for babies with a poor sucking reflex. Silicone teats are harder and longer-lasting but more expensive. There were concerns raised in the 1980s about nitrosamines contained in latex teats. Nitrosamines are known to cause cancer in animals. Silicone teats contain far fewer nitrosamines than latex teats, so if you are worried about them, choose silicone.

- Different teats have different flows – the speed at which milk comes out of the bottle when your baby suckles. Follow the maker's guidelines on which is the appropriate flow for your baby – slow, medium or fast. It will usually depend on age, but sometimes your baby might prefer a faster or a slower flow. You'll need to change teats as your baby gets older.

- There are also variflow teats, which vary the flow depending on how hard your baby sucks, allowing her to feed faster when she is more hungry.

- Change teats every couple of months or when you can see they have scratches in order to reduce the chance of bacteria growing.

A good latch

- Your baby's lips should be open wide, touching the base of the teat all the way around, with the top lip visible and the bottom lip rolled outwards.

- Just as with breastfeeding, a good part of the teat should be in your baby's mouth, not just the nipple.

- Your baby's jaw should move when she is sucking and you should hear swallowing.

Optional extras

- **A bottle warmer**, which can be useful in the middle of the night for heating up bottles but can take up a lot of room in a kitchen. Bottles can be just as easily warmed in some hot water or, very carefully and with a good shake afterwards, in a microwave.

- **A powder dispenser and thermos** for carrying hot, boiled water when you are out and about if you are making up powdered formula.

Alternatives to bottles

Supplemental nursing systems

If you wish to continue feeding your baby at the breast but need to supplement with formula, expressed milk or donor milk, a supplemental nursing system (SNS) allows you to do this without introducing a bottle. It consists of a bottle worn around the mother's neck and attached to a very thin tube that sits next to the nipple, allowing a baby to suck on the breast and the tube at the same time.

If you are trying to build your supply, this can be a great way of ensuring that your baby gets what she needs via the bottle, while stimulating milk production by sucking. It can also be a good way to continue the closeness of breastfeeding. However, if you have underlying issues that have caused a low milk supply or your baby has her own difficulties feeding, it is not necessarily a long-term solution to the problem.

If you would like to use an SNS, it is best to speak to a breastfeeding counsellor to talk through your feeding issues and figure out whether they might be helped by using this system.

Nursettes

Nursettes is the name given to a combined pack of ready-to-feed formula with a disposable teat. They come ready to use – you only need to attach the disposable teat to the disposable bottle.

They are a good option for newborns, especially in hospital, because the pack is fully sterile, requiring no sterilisation of bottles or preparation of formula. However, they are very expensive so not a viable long-term solution, and most supermarkets and pharmacies don't carry them. It is possible to buy them over the internet.

3 Sterilising

I'm not here to lie to you – sterilising bottles is a pain. It requires forethought, organisation and a whole bunch of equipment that clogs up your cupboards. Anyone who says that bottle-feeding is the easy way out has never had to prepare a nappy bag for an exclusively formula-fed baby on a day out. Talk about military organisation.

Sterilising is, however, an essential part of preparing bottles. Not only can nasty bacteria grow in powdered and reconstituted formula, they can also thrive in feeding equipment. You may have noticed that American websites advise that sterilising is not necessary and bottles can simply be put in a hot wash in the dishwasher. Current British official advice is that *all feeding equipment should be sterilised at least until your baby is six months old.*

With all of that said, once you get the hang of sterilising, it's fine – and, after all, forethought, organisation and equipment are all standard-issue skills needed in modern motherhood.

Sterilising equipment and how to sterilise

There are a number of ways you can sterilise bottles. Regardless of which way you choose, the first steps are the same:

- Wash your hands. This is so important. Washing your hands should become a reflex action to any formula-feeding parent, any time you touch anything to do with your baby's feeds.
- Unscrew all the parts of the bottle and wash them separately in hot, soapy water. They can also be washed in a dishwasher. Even if you wash in a dishwasher, they still need to be sterilised – but sterilising

doesn't work if there are bits of old milk in the bottle. It's a good idea to thoroughly rinse your baby's bottles as soon as she finishes drinking them. You can then do your full wash and sterilisation once a day.

Steam sterilisers

These are large sterilisers that fit a number of bottles, teats, collars and lids as well as other equipment such as breast pumps. They are easy, fast and thorough. Simply follow the manufacturer's instructions. The downside is that they take up a lot of bench space.

Microwave steam sterilisers

These are another version of the steam steriliser that fits a number of bottles and teats and are an excellent choice if you have a microwave. Follow the manufacturer's instructions, and the above instructions for keeping bottles sterile.

Chemical sterilising

It's possible to buy tablets or fluids that you put into water with bottles and other equipment to sterilise. This is a good option if you're travelling, but it takes longer than steam sterilisers. Bottles need to be fully submerged and then rinsed with previously boiled water, which makes the process more complicated.

Sterilising by boiling

The old-school way to sterilise is to completely submerge bottles and teats in water, cover the pan with a lid, bring it to a rolling boil, and then leave the bottles and teats submerged in the pan with the lid on until needed. This is the least convenient way as the bottles have a tendency to pop out of the water, and most waters will leave some chalky residue on the bottles. Avoid this method if you can.

Sterile rules

When using a steam or microwave steam steriliser you can use the tongs provided to reassemble the bottle immediately, including replacing the bottle lid to stop the teat being exposed to the air, and store the assembled bottle on your countertop. Alternatively, you can leave the bottles in the steriliser with its lid on tightly until you need them. Bottles sterilised this way remain sterile for about 24 hours.

Remember: coming into contact with anything that isn't sterile, including air, gives the bottle the opportunity to pick up germs.

If you don't use the bottle, you will need to re-sterilise it 24 hours later.

How long to keep sterilising?

Official advice is to sterilise until your baby is around six months old. Many people point out that, because babies older than six months are picking up germs as they crawl around and are eating unsterile solids, sterilising bottles is unnecessary. However, because bottles are ideal breeding grounds for bacteria due to their warm, wet environments, there is good reason to continue sterilisation until your baby weans from the bottle. This is a personal choice, but there is no harm in prolonging sterilisation for as long as you feel it is beneficial.

4 Preparing a feed

It is essential that you prepare and store formula safely in order to minimise the chance of your baby becoming ill. The following guidelines about preparing feeds are designed to minimise the risk of contamination while preserving the nutrients of formula, and are based on the WHO's recommendations.

The golden rules

- Wash your hands before touching anything to do with your baby's feeds.
- Make up each feed fresh when possible.
- Throw out unused feeds no later than two hours after you have made them up. Never put a half-finished bottle back in the fridge for later use.
- Be assiduous about cleaning and sterilising bottles.

Preparing ready-to-feed formula

- Wash your hands and clean the area where you will prepare the bottle. It's a good idea to keep a little area of your kitchen bench exclusively for preparing bottles, to minimise the risk of contamination from food.
- Open the carton and pour the necessary amount into your sterilised bottle. Immediately put the rest of the used carton into a fridge that is 5° Celsius or lower. Put it at the back of the fridge where the temperature is more stable, and definitely not in the door. You need to use this carton within 24 hours of opening, so write the time you opened it on the carton, otherwise you are guaranteed to forget. It's fine to mix from different cartons, as long as none of them has been opened for longer than 24 hours.

- Give the bottle at your baby's preferred temperature. Most babies are fine with room temperature formula, which is much more convenient for you. It's a myth that babies need formula warmed to body temperature.
- Throw away any used formula no later than two hours after you prepared the bottle and immediately rinse the bottle and teat thoroughly, ready to be washed and sterilised later.

Preparing powdered formula

- Wash your hands and clean the area where you will prepare the feed.
- Throw out any water in the kettle, put in at least a litre of fresh water and boil it. Never re-boil water that has already been sitting in the kettle. Allow the water to cool for no more than 30 minutes, which will let it drop to about 70° Celsius, which is the temperature the WHO and UK Department of Health recommend all powdered formula be prepared at in order to kill any salmonella or *Cronobacter sakazakii* that may be present in the powder. If the water is still boiling, it will destroy some of the vitamins and minerals in the formula.
- Unscrew the collar, teat and lid of your sterilised bottle all together, and place them upside down on your clean work surface so that no part of the teat touches the surface.
- Pour the amount of water in for the feed that you think you baby will need. (See page 190 for guidelines on how much to feed.) It is essential that you *put the water in first* to make sure that formula is not over- or under-concentrated.
- Using clean hands, measure out into the bottle the number of *level* scoops of formula that the manufacturer recommends for the amount of water you are using. Most formula tins come with a built-in leveller. If you need to use a knife, use a clean one to scrape off a level scoop every time and don't put it back in the tin or reuse it. *Never compact down the formula in the scoop.* Different formulas come with different scoops, so only use the one provided. It is very important to always use exactly the amount of levelled-off formula specified by the manufacturer. Putting in too much or too little for the amount of water you're using is dangerous for your baby.
- Screw the collar, teat and lid together back on, and give the bottle a good shake to dissolve all the formula. Don't overshake or you'll get too many bubbles, which can pass into your baby's tummy.

- Cool the formula down by running the bottle under a cold tap, making sure not to get the lid wet, or by putting the bottom in cold or iced water. It will take a couple of minutes to cool down sufficiently to give to your baby. Test it by putting a few drops on your wrist. It's the right temperature when you can almost not feel it – that means it's body temperature. Most babies will also happily take bottles that are at room temperature or even cold.
- Give the bottle, and throw out any unused formula after two hours. Rinse the bottle and teat.

Feeding during the night

If your baby is on a regular feeding schedule and you can anticipate when she will need a feed 30 minutes before she starts crying for one, the above guidelines are fine. However, in the middle of the night it is obviously not feasible to sit around waiting for water to cool for 30 minutes while a hungry baby wails beside you.

While WHO guidelines say that preparing each feed as needed is the preferred method, they also say that where this is not possible, feeds can be prepared up to 24 hours in advance and left in the fridge.[1] This is what you will most likely want to do for feeds in the middle of the night. In this case, you need to follow the steps below:

- Prepare the number of feeds you will need as per the instructions above, making sure you allow the water to cool to no less than 70° Celsius before adding the powder. You might also want to prepare your baby's first feed of the day if she demands a bottle as soon as she wakes up.
- Put the made-up bottles at the back of a fridge that is no warmer than 5° Celsius.
- As needed, take out a bottle and reheat it either by running it under the hot water tap or by putting it in a bottle warmer. WHO and Department of Health guidelines say that microwaves shouldn't be used to reheat bottles because they can create 'hot spots' in the milk that can burn a baby's mouth. However, the anecdotal experience of many parents suggests that it is fine to reheat bottles to room temperature in a microwave (after removing the teat and lid) and then give the bottle a good shake to even out the heat.
- Feed your baby, discard any unused feed and rinse the teat and bottle.

Feeding out and about

By far the easiest way to give bottles of formula while out and about is to bring sterilised bottles and cartons of ready-to-feed formula that you can open and give as needed.

Alternatively, you can bring prepared bottles of formula in a refrigerated bag with an ice brick, though this is often impractical as it's difficult to keep the bottles below the required 5° Celsius.

The third option is to mix powdered formula at your destination. It's possible to buy formula powder dispensers into which you measure the required amount of formula before you leave home. You then simply tip it into the bottle of water when you're out. You can bring a thermos of freshly boiled water with you, to pour into your bottles on site.

A common dilemma – safety versus practicality

Many parents prepare bottles in another way, which is very practical but not recommended by the WHO or Department of Health. Following this method, enough water is boiled for the day's feeds then poured into sterilised bottles that are closed and capped in order to preserve sterility. The bottles are then left to cool to room temperature or put in the fridge. Parents then simply add the powder to the bottles as needed.

This method has a number of upsides: it's convenient because there is no waiting for bottles to cool or water to boil; the bottles of water remain sterile until the powder is added; and none of the micronutrients in the formula are damaged by water that is too hot. The downside is that if there are dangerous bacteria in the powder, they won't be killed off as you're not putting the formula in at the recommended 70° Celsius.

While the risk of *Cronobacter* being present in your formula powder is very, very small, it is still a risk, and a small number of babies are infected with the bacteria every year. It may interest you to know that even though British guidelines don't recommend formula be made with room temperature water, Australian health guidelines say it is fine, because health bodies there believe the risk of *Cronobacter* being present in Australian formula tins is negligible.

We can't tell you whether this method is okay; all we can do is present you with the facts and let you make your own decision. As with every parenting choice you make, you need to weigh up the possible risks and benefits to see whether it is right for you family.

Which water?

Boiled tap water is most commonly used for making up bottles, and if you live somewhere with a safe water supply it is a perfectly safe option as long as it's boiled. It needs to be boiled because regular tap water contains bacteria that are fine for adults, but not for babies. This is why you should *never use unboiled water from the tap*.

Lead

In certain cities such as London, which have old lead pipes in houses, there is a greater risk of tap water containing a higher level of lead than is recommended. Too much lead affects babies' brain development. If you live somewhere with old water pipes, *always run your tap for a minute* before you fill the kettle. This allows water that has been sitting in the pipes, potentially absorbing more lead, to run out, leaving you with fresher water. While a standard domestic pitcher water filter reduces some impurities, most don't do a lot for lead.

Bottled water

Generally, you should not use bottled mineral water for preparing formula as it usually contains levels of sodium and sulphate that are too high for babies. Check on the label – if there is less than 200 mg of sodium (also written as Na) per litre, and less than 250 mg of sulphate (also written as SO or SO4) per litre it should be okay to use. You will still need to boil it, though.[2]

Purified water can be used as long as it contains safe levels of sodium and sulphate and has been boiled.

Fluoride in water

Fluoride protects against dental cavities but too much fluoride can lead to brown mottling of tooth enamel (fluorosis). Whether fluoride is added to your water supply depends on where you live – most countries in Europe no longer add fluoride, but many local authorities in the UK, Australia and the US still do. If you live in a fluoridated area, as long as your local water authority is following guidelines, the fluoride consumption of your baby should be within guidelines, but it is up to you to check. The very upper limit for fluoride intake for babies up to six months is 0.7 mg per day,[3] but it's better for babies to consume less. Breastfed babies consume about 0.01 mg of fluoride a day and that is considered adequate. Powdered formula already contains some fluoride, though most fluoride exposure for formula-fed babies comes from the water used to prepare it.

Ready-to-feed formulas are generally prepared with demineralised tap water and fall within safe fluoride levels.

Pitcher filters don't remove fluoride, though other, more expensive filter systems do.

5 Feeding

Feeding is much more than just giving your baby the nutrients she needs to thrive; it's an important way of showing love, building trust and developing the bond that will become the foundation of her psychological well-being. However, because formula-feeding parents are given so little information, many don't know that there is so much more to formula-feeding than just 'giving a bottle'.

Here we give you not only the nuts and bolts of how to give a feed and how much, but how to do it to promote closeness and bonding. Hopefully, by using some of the suggestions here you'll be able to ease any guilt you may feel about using a bottle. The elation of nourishing your precious baby isn't only for breastfeeding mums, and you'll find that the more you put into each feed, the more you and your baby get out of it.

Reading your baby's hunger cues

Health authorities recommend feeding your baby on demand, whether you are breastfeeding or bottle-feeding. You should always be led by your baby's hunger cues – never try to feed her if she doesn't appear to be hungry. Responding to hunger cues promptly helps to build up trust and a good bond between you and your baby, which is another reason why feeding on demand is recommended. (That said, some sleepy new babies may need to be woken for feeds. If they eagerly take a bottle once they have woken up then they are hungry.)

You *can* overfeed a baby, and it is easier to overfeed a bottle-fed baby than a breastfed one. Your baby knows how much food she needs, so trust her – offer her milk when she seems hungry, and stop when she seems like she's had enough.

If you're coming to bottle-feeding a couple of months into your baby's life, you'll know how to read her hunger cues. If you're starting out with a newborn, here are a few signs your baby wants a feed:

- 'rooting around' with her mouth as though looking for a nipple
- opening her mouth wide and sticking out her tongue
- sucking on her fist
- sucking on your clean finger when you put it into her mouth
- moving her arms and legs around
- starting to fuss
- crying – this is a late hunger signal and it's better to offer a feed before your baby gets to this stage if you can.

Obviously, some of these signs are also saying 'I've done a poo' or 'I have gas' and it can be nerve-wracking trying to decipher your baby's language when you're first beginning. However, we promise that you will soon learn which signs mean 'I'm hungry'. You have nothing to lose from offering a bottle – she won't take it if she doesn't want it. Just remember never to force a feed.

Bottle-feeding – a basic guide

You'll soon figure out the ways that work for you and your baby, but here's how to get started.

- Make sure your baby is awake and ready to feed. Trying to feed a sleepy baby is a frustrating experience for both of you.
- Get yourself in a relaxed position where you can cradle your baby closely to you. A natural way is with her head in the crook of your arm, just as you would if you were breastfeeding. Her body should be held at a 45 degree angle or greater. This is for two reasons: if she's lying flat it's easier for milk to drip into her mouth, making it more difficult to co-ordinate sucking and swallowing; also, a more upright angle reduces the risk of ear infection. Another position is holding her head in your hand at a 90 degree angle to you, so you are facing each other.
- Take the bottle and gently tickle her upper lip, nose or cheek with it to encourage her to open her mouth wide.
- Gently put the teat in, allowing her to grasp it with her tongue and jaw and start sucking. Don't force it in. If she doesn't accept it, that's

a sign she's not hungry. If she's hungry she'll start sucking with gusto.

- Make sure that the nipple is completely filled with milk so that she's not sucking down any air.
- Check that she has a good latch: her lips should be open wide, with the top lip visible and the bottom lip rolled outwards and touching the base of the teat all the way around. A good part of the teat should be in her mouth, not just the nipple, and her jaw should move when she is sucking. (Her bottom lip should always be rolled outwards and her top lip always visible. If they aren't, you can correct the latch manually with your thumb and finger, but if you're finding you repeatedly need to do this, you probably have the wrong teat.)
- She'll need little breaks during the feed so watch her for signals. (Babies take breaks when they breastfeed so they need to when bottle-feeding too.) As she slows down the sucking a little, try removing the bottle. This gives her a natural gap in the feed and helps to prevent overfeeding. You need to remove the bottle so that excess milk doesn't drip into her mouth when she doesn't want it.
- You can use this gap to give her a little burp: sit her upright with your hand supporting her chin and rub her back, or put her over your shoulder. You don't need to pat her vigorously – a gentle rub should generally do it.
- Once the little break is over, offer her the bottle again by again rubbing it on her upper lip, cheek or nose. If she doesn't take it, that means she's had enough. If she's hardly had any, you can give it a rest for 10 or 15 minutes and offer it to her again after that.
- Listen for her swallowing – it should sound effortless and happen after every one or two sucks.
- It's important to swap arms, just as you would swap breasts if you were breastfeeding. This helps to develop her eyes equally.
- Be led by your baby, not the bottle. Never try to get her to finish it if she doesn't want to.
- Don't let your baby fall asleep with a bottle. Not only will you regret this when you need to train her to fall asleep on her own later on, once she has teeth they need to be cleaned after her last feed of the day.
- Never, ever prop a bottle up. Bottles should always be held by you, or your baby when she is old enough.

- Bottle-feeds usually end up taking between 10 and 20 minutes. Much slower than that and you could either be using the wrong teat or have a slower flow than is needed, but be led by your baby on this.

Some signs your baby has had enough

- Pushing her tongue up to push out the teat
- Turning her head away
- Gagging or crying
- Generally looking uncomfortable
- Arching her back
- Breaking eye contact and looking uninterested.

Burping and spitting up

You don't need to spend hours burping your baby with violent pats, but if she has swallowed some air it needs to come out. Do it for a few minutes after a feed.

It's completely normal for a little bit of the feed to be regurgitated, so be prepared with a cloth over your shoulder. Regular, larger vomits are something that may need to be discussed with your health professional.

If your baby appears to be uncomfortable during or after a feed, either crying constantly, arching her back or wriggling around, this could be the sign of a more serious problem such as reflux or allergy. This should be discussed with a doctor or nurse.

Feeding with love

We cannot emphasise enough how important it is to be a sensitive, 'present' parent when you give your baby a bottle. Babies benefit emotionally and most likely cognitively from being fed in a loving and close way. Feeding, whether at the breast or from the bottle, is a great opportunity for you and your baby to get to know each other and bond.

You don't need to spend every feed gazing into your baby's eyes, but, equally, don't treat every feed as an opportunity to catch up on

Downton Abbey and Facebook. Feeding with love benefits not only your baby but you as well – you will find feeding much more rewarding, particularly if you are grieving over not breastfeeding.

Some ways to feed with love

- Respond promptly to your baby's hunger cues, and get her bottle before she is in a full-on wail.
- Look into your baby's eyes – the big advantage of bottle-feeding is that it gives your baby an easier position to be able to look at you properly.
- Hold her close.
- Sing and talk to your baby.
- Feed her *skin to skin* as often as you feel comfortable doing so. As discussed in Chapter 2, skin-to-skin contact releases oxytocin, 'the love hormone', which helps promote feelings of mutual closeness. I used to do this a lot with my daughter and we both loved it.
- Try to restrict feeding to you and your partner. Having a regular provider of food helps to build your baby's trust in you, and helps to forge a bond. The occasional feed by someone else is okay, but you and your partner should be the main bottle-givers.
- As your baby gets older she will be able to hold her own bottle, but she will still enjoy the closeness of a cuddle, and so will you. You'll miss it when she's too independent to spend those quiet moments snuggling, so make the most of them while you can!

How much milk?

There are so many different guidelines for how much milk your baby needs. It can be very confusing, particularly when different brands of formula recommend different amounts.

The real answer is that your baby needs what she tells you she needs. Infants naturally regulate their intake, and you need to learn to read the signs they give you about when they are hungry and when they're not. However, I realise that's not remotely helpful when you're starting out with bottle-feeding, so here's something more concrete:

The Royal College of Nursing advises parents to feed on demand, and as a guideline says that newborns between the ages of one week and three months need 150 ml per kilogram of body weight per day. They advise that most full-term babies will need to be fed every two to four hours (closer to every two when they're first born). Because newborn babies have tiny stomachs, they will gradually increase their intake from about 20 to 30 ml/kg on the first day of life to 150 ml/kg by seven days.[1] Once a baby hits three months, she needs a little less – 120 ml/kg/day – and once solids are introduced at around six months she'll need even less.

If you are topping up after breastfeeds, it's obviously much harder to give guidelines – you'll need to be led more by your baby's cues. Try starting with 20 to 30 ml per feed and take it from there.

Guidelines for formula consumption[2]

Age	Number of feeds/ how much	ml/kg/day	Suggested total daily consumption
0–7 days	8–10 feeds, 10 ml/ feed, gradually increasing to 50 ml/ feed	20–30 ml/kg/ day, gradually increasing to 150 ml/kg/day	70–105 ml gradually increasing to up to 525 ml
7 days – 2 weeks	7–8 feeds/day, 60–70 ml/feed	150 ml/kg/day	420–560 ml
2 weeks – 2 months	6–7 feeds/day, 75–105 ml/feed	150 ml/kg/day	450–735 ml
2–3 months	5–6 feeds/day, 105–180 ml/feed	150 ml/kg/day	525–1080 ml
3–4 months	5 feeds/day, 180–210 ml/feed	150 ml/kg/day	900–1050 ml
4–5 months	5 feeds/day, 180–210 ml/feed	120 ml/kg/day	900–1050 ml
Around 6 months	4 feeds/day, 210–240 ml/feed	120 ml/kg/day	840–960 ml

Remember: this is a guideline only. You'll soon find your own way, and you will likely find that your baby regularly takes more feeds at some times than others.

By six months of age, your baby will have started eating solids and will gradually need less and less milk, as solids start to provide a greater proportion of her nutritional needs.

By around 1 year, when a healthy baby can move from formula onto cow's milk, she can consume up to 400 ml of formula divided how you like, perhaps split between two small bottles and a larger bottle before bedtime.

Changing teats

As your baby grows, you will need to change teat sizes on the bottle, to allow for a faster flow. Be guided by your baby on this. If she is sucking hard and appears to be getting frustrated with the bottle, she may need a faster-flowing one. If she is spluttering and gagging, she'll probably need a slower teat. Manufacturers give indications on the box about the appropriate age for each teat.

Moving from formula to cow's milk

As discussed on page 168, current health guidelines suggest that formula-fed babies move to whole cow's milk once they reach their first birthday, with no need to move to a follow-on formula.

Don't try to switch from one day to the next. What's easier is gradually replacing a little of the formula in your baby's bottle with cow's milk over a week or two, so she gets used to the new taste.

If your baby really loves her formula and flat out refuses cow's milk, you have two choices – either you can continue to pay the extra expense of formula, or you can just forgo milk altogether, making sure she gets her calcium needs met through cheese, yoghurt and milk in cooking. If you choose the former, you can have another go at swapping in a few months.

When to stop bottle-feeding

Most child health nurses will tell you that you should move from bottles to sippy cups or cups when your baby turns one. Most bottle-feeding parents will tell you that babies continue to enjoy a bedtime bottle until they're 2 or older.

The push to switch comes from the risk of dental cavities, which is greater in bottle-fed babies than in breastfed ones. However, this risk comes from allowing milk (which is high in natural sugars) to pool around a baby's teeth, not from the bottle itself. If you properly clean your baby's teeth *after* her last feed of the day and practise proper oral hygiene (see below), you have no reason to be worried, and your baby can continue to enjoy her bedtime bottle for as long as she's interested. For me and my daughter, that was about 18 months.

Remember, though, that by the age of one the great majority of your baby's calories should be coming from food, not milk, so if she is still having four or more large bottles a day you will need to cut down.

Oral hygiene

Whether you are breastfeeding or bottle-feeding, as soon as your baby gets a tooth, it needs to be cleaned. Bottles get a lot of bad press when it comes to rotting teeth, but as long as you make sure you clean your baby's teeth before she goes to bed, but *after* her last bottle of the day, you have no reason to be worried.

A few tips:

- If your baby has teeth and is still having a bottle in the middle of the night, you can clean her teeth when she wakes up in the morning.
- You can start cleaning first teeth with a muslin wrapped around your finger, and when she has a few more teeth, move on to using a toothbrush.
- Avoid letting your baby or toddler wander around with a bottle or sippy cup of milk for prolonged periods of time – this increases the likelihood of cavities. If your child refuses to give up the comfort bottle, change it to water.

Combining breast and bottle

Many mothers will end up combining breastfeeding and bottle-feeding, or 'mixed feeding' as it's generally known. This can be for a host of reasons including issues with milk supply, work, sleep, medication or emotions. Mixed feeding can mean either topping up with formula after regular breastfeeds or replacing some feeds with formula.

Detailed instructions on how to mixed-feed are beyond the scope of this book, but many breastfeeding books have guides on the subject that can help you.

You do need to be aware that if you are breastfeeding and are considering introducing some formula, your breast milk supply will likely be affected. If you want to continue breastfeeding alongside bottle-feeding, it's best to wait for a couple of months until you have fully established your supply, and your baby has got the hang of the latch. However, in reality, we know that many women introduce formula before that.

This also clashes a little with advice on when is best to introduce a bottle so that a baby doesn't reject either the bottle or the breast. Opinions on this vary widely, from two to eight weeks. One way to bring in a bottle without overly affecting your breast milk supply is to express a feed for your partner to give.

Some breastfeeding counsellors strongly advise against giving a bottle, even of expressed milk, because they say it creates 'nipple confusion' – when a baby has trouble switching from bottle to breast. Others say nipple confusion is a scare tactic used to frighten women away from bottle-feeding, and if a baby rejected the breast after taking a bottle the real issue is an underlying breastfeeding problem.

If you need to supplement with formula in the first week of life while waiting for your milk to come in, you could use other options – these include a syringe, a small cup, a finger or a supplemental nursing system. It's best to speak to a healthcare professional about these.

Ultimately, many families successfully mix breastfeeding and formula-feeding, and it can be a practical way to continue to give your baby the benefits of breast milk while working within the constraints of your life and your family.

6 Switching from breast to bottle

Getting babies to accept a bottle can be one of the biggest hurdles for bottle-feeding families. It can also be easy as pie – no one knows how your baby will react to a bottle until you try. While many readers of this book will already be well down the bottle path, for those who are stopping breastfeeding for the first time, here are a few hints on how to introduce a bottle.[1]

When? (If you have a choice)

If you know that you are going to be using a bottle eventually, it's a good idea to introduce it early, say at three or four weeks, with one feed of expressed breast milk or formula a day. Some breastfeeding advocates will warn you against this by saying that it can create nipple confusion but many experienced midwives say nipple confusion is actually a symptom of deeper breastfeeding problems, rather than of problems caused by the bottle. Personally, I first introduced a bottle as a regular part of my baby's feeding routine when she was six days old, and we continued happily mixed-feeding for seven weeks, with her eagerly taking both breast and bottle. Anecdotally, it seems that waiting until a baby is two months or older makes bottle rejection more likely, though not guaranteed.

If you haven't introduced a bottle yet and your baby is a little older but you know you have a deadline coming up, such as returning to work, do start trying a couple of weeks ahead of time, just in case it doesn't go to plan.

The first feed

Just as with breastfeeding, both your baby and you need to learn how to bottle-feed, so the key thing to remember is to be patient. If you've been breastfeeding for a long time without using a bottle, it is entirely to be expected that your baby won't be that keen to start. Try not to get stressed as your baby will pick up on your cues.

- Choose a time for the first bottle when your baby is not tired and isn't too hungry – a snack time in between main breastfeeds is good.
- Warm the milk to body temperature. Babies will happily accept room temperature or cold bottles eventually, but it's a good idea to keep everything as familiar as possible until a bottle is well established.
- If you are able to express milk, try that instead of formula for the same reason.
- Hold your baby close as you normally would. We would normally suggest feeding skin to skin, but you don't want to confuse your baby by having your breast there and not using it, so until you have both got the hang of the bottle it's best to keep clothes on.
- Don't shove the bottle in your baby's mouth – look at 'Bottle-feeding – a basic guide' on page 186.

What if your baby consistently refuses a bottle?

It's time to bring in the big guns – daddy, grandmother, mother-in-law, etc. Many a mother complains of babies steadfastly refusing to take a bottle from them, but happily taking one from another family member. You may find physically leaving the house helps too, both so that you're not upset and so that your baby doesn't sense that you're there and howl until you unclip your nursing bra.

Get an experienced bottle-feeder to help you. Stay calm and keep trying!

Stopping the production of breast milk

If you are switching to bottles altogether, it's preferable to do so gradually, if you can, to allow your body to adjust naturally to producing less milk. This reduces not only uncomfortable breast pressure but also the chances of blocked ducts and mastitis.

One way to reduce discomfort is to give the first half of all feeds with formula, and then finish with breast milk, so you are regularly emptying your breasts but your baby is gradually demanding less volume.

If you need to stop suddenly, your breasts will feel very uncomfortable if you had a good milk supply. You can reduce the pressure by hand-expressing a little in the shower (or whenever you feel you're going to burst!). Pumping and breastfeeding will only encourage production again, so try to avoid these.

7 Common bottle-feeding side effects and problems

Like anything to do with babies, when bottle-feeding you'll run up against problems, have a million questions and want to tear your hair out sometimes. This is all part of the ride, but to help a little we've collated a few of the most common side effects and problems you're likely to encounter with formula-feeding.

For answers to those questions we haven't addressed, make sure you go online and join a support group, or, even better, create your own face-to-face support group of bottle-feeding parents. Many heads are better than one.

Hard poos and constipation

Formula-fed babies tend to poo only once a day, or even less frequently, and the poo is generally harder than the poo of breastfed babies. It smells different too – this is completely normal. It is normal for both breastfed and formula-fed babies to grunt and go a little red in the face when they are doing a poo. It doesn't mean they are constipated.

True constipation is when poo is hard and dry, and it is often caused by dehydration. It can look like rabbit droppings. It is rare in babies under three months, even formula-fed ones. In addition to hard and dry poo, babies will be very uncomfortable or even in pain when pooing. You may find little cracks around her anus. Watch for blood in her stools.

How to manage it

- Check you are making the formula correctly, not putting in too little water, and always putting the water in first.
- Gently massage your baby's tummy by rubbing it in a clockwise direction. Stop if it seems to be causing pain.
- Move her legs in a cycling motion. This moves her stomach muscles, which then stimulates the intestines to move too.
- Add a little extra water to her bottle. This can make the poo softer, but remember to add only a little. If your baby is normally drinking 150 ml per bottle, for example, try adding an extra 10 ml and see if that helps. You need to be very careful with this, though – diluting formula much more than this can be dangerous because it risks babies not getting the essential levels of potassium and sodium.
- Give some cooled, boiled water in between feeds. Again, only a little, especially if your baby is still small.
- Consider changing formula. A 100% whey formula might be more easily digested.
- See a doctor if these approaches don't work.

Ear infection

Formula-fed babies are more prone to ear infection than breastfed babies. While some of this is likely because formula lacks the anti-infective properties that are found in breast milk, it could also be down to the way you are feeding your baby.

How to manage it

- Always feed your baby at a 45 degree angle or greater. If you feed your baby horizontally, the Eustachian tube – the tube that connects the back of the throat to the middle ear – is more flat, which allows germs to travel more easily from the throat to the ear. Keep your baby upright for a little while after a feed too.

Colic or wind

Colic is an imprecise term used to describe continued, unexplained crying. It's usually presumed to arise from pains in the tummy; however, many experienced midwives say it's simply a normal part of being a baby. It can be very distressing for parents who naturally want to fix whatever is wrong, but don't know how.

How to manage it

- Because formula is more difficult to digest than breast milk, your baby may show some discomfort after a bottle, including pulling her knees up to her chest, squirming and crying. If this continues and you are worried about it, then by all means try a different formula. Remember, though, don't change formulas too often as this can cause more tummy upsets.
- A lot of parents try Infacol and gripe water too. Infacol is an anti-foaming agent that is given via a little dropper. In adults it has been shown to allow them to pass wind more easily; however, there is little robust evidence that it works for children, nor is there for gripe water. By all means try them though – some parents swear by them.

It's normal for babies to pass wind regularly and loudly. You may find that if you have been breastfeeding and then switched to formula she passes wind more often. As long as she doesn't appear to be in pain, this isn't a problem. If the wind appears to cause pain, you might like to try massaging her tummy and moving her legs in a cycling motion to help ease the wind out. Again, try a different formula if discomfort persists and see a doctor if you are worried.

Reflux

Reflux isn't caused by formula; it is a condition where the muscle ring that seals the stomach off from the oesophagus hasn't properly developed yet, allowing the acidic contents of the stomach to regurgitate back up. It is quite common in babies – some estimates suggest that as many as one in five babies suffer from reflux. Symptoms include significant or persistent vomiting, which can lead to weight loss or failure to thrive, discomfort after feeds, including excessive crying and irritability, arching, stiffening, difficulty breathing, a hoarse cry and a chronic cough.

It is possible to buy anti-reflux formulas that have been thickened and have a higher casein ratio; however, they are not recommended by the European Society of Paediatric Gastroenterology, Hepatology and Nutrition.

It is normal for babies to regurgitate some milk after a feed. This is not reflux.

If you are worried that your baby may have reflux, including silent reflux (where milk regurgitates only into the oesophagus without coming out of the mouth), you should speak to a doctor. There are a number of treatments available.

Cow's milk allergy

Allergies aren't caused by formula, but if your baby has a cow's milk allergy or intolerance then she will have a lot of difficulty digesting regular formula. Around one in 50 babies is allergic to cow's milk and dairy products. If your baby has previously been breastfed, the allergy may not have been obvious.

The symptoms of allergy are diverse and may occur immediately after taking formula or several days afterwards. They include hives, eczema, vomiting, diarrhoea, wheezing and anaphylaxis.

See your doctor to get a diagnosis of cow's milk allergy or intolerance. For a milk-allergic baby, an extensively hydrolysed formula is the first choice. Soya formulas and amino acid-based formulas are other options, but all should be discussed with a doctor. A significant minority of babies who are allergic to cow's milk will also be allergic to soya.

Resources

Here is a small selection of sources of trustworthy information and help.

Bottle-feeding support

www.bottlebabies.org: A wonderful support group for bottle families, and a great source of information and practical help.

www.fearlessformulafeeder.com: Provides advocacy for bottle-feeding families, support and intelligent comments on feeding issues.

incredibleinfant.com: An American-based blog that regularly has tips on formula-feeding.

There is an increasing number of localised bottle-feeding support groups on Facebook. Look for one in your area.

Formula companies also provide telephone and online information services staffed by trained midwives and nutritionists.

Breastfeeding support

www.breastfeedingnetwork.org.uk: Breastfeeding support network that runs drop-in centres and telephone counselling.

abm.me.uk: The Association of Breastfeeding Mothers runs a breastfeeding helpline and has contacts for local support groups.

www.lcgb.org: Lactation Consultants of Great Britain has contacts for public and private lactation consultants.

Formula composition and help choosing a formula

www.firststepsnutrition.org: This British-based charity provides the most thorough, regularly updated, independent information on formula available, while maintaining a strong pro-breastfeeding stance. A must visit for anyone wishing to cut through formula company marketing when choosing a formula.

Safe bottle preparation

www.unicef.org.uk/Documents/Baby_Friendly/Leaflets/guide_to_bottle_feeding.pdf: Easy-to-read guidelines from UNICEF – with pictures!

www.nhs.uk/conditions/pregnancy-and-baby/pages/making-up-infant-formula.aspx: Guidelines from the NHS.

www.who.int/foodsafety/publications/micro/pif_guidelines.pdf: A very comprehensive guide from the WHO intended for nurses and parents.

Advice for mothers with specific breastfeeding problems

www.bfar.org: Breastfeeding after breast and nipple surgery.

www.llli.org/llleaderweb/lv/lviss2-3-2009p4.html: Good information on insufficient glandular tissue (IGT) or hypoplasia.

d-mer.org: Information on this rare and only recently discovered condition.

Advice on babies with feeding problems

www.cumbria.nhs.uk/ProfessionalZone/MedicinesManagement/Guidelines/Infant-formula-milk-prescribing-guidelines.pdf: This page is intended for clinicians but it is the best page we have seen on diagnosing and treating cow's milk allergy and intolerance and lactose intolerance.

www.reflux.org.au: Support and information on reflux.

www.nhs.uk/conditions/tongue-tie: A good page on tongue tie, with good links including a list of hospitals that provide tongue-tie surgery.

Postnatal depression and anxiety

www.postpartumprogress.com: The world's most widely read blog on perinatal mental health problems.

www.pni.org.uk: Information and peer support.

www.cope.org.au: An Australian centre of excellence for perinatal mental health, with an international focus.

Scientific research into breastfeeding and infant health

www.ncbi.nlm.nih.gov/pmc: PubMed Central is a free full-text archive of biomedical and life sciences journal literature maintained by the US government. Many journal articles are published here, though often journals restrict access to their latest articles. A great place to read the research for yourself.

www.thecochranelibrary.com: A wonderful collection of systematic reviews of health research. One of the highest-quality sources of science information on the internet.

www.mommadata.blogspot.co.uk: The blog of Polly Palumbo, PhD. She dissects studies, and the media's reporting of those studies, on a wide variety of parenting topics, and cuts through the crap with style and warmth.

emedicine.medscape.com: Gives very useful, comprehensive and (mostly) understandable reviews of common medical problems, including diagnosis and management of infant reflux (see the section on reflux).

Recommended books on feeding and/or motherhood

Barston, S., *Bottled Up: How the Way We Feed Babies Has Come to Define Motherhood, and Why it Shouldn't*, Berkeley: University of California Press, 2012.

Douglas, S. and M. Michaels, *The Mommy Myth: The Idealization of Motherhood and How It Has Undermined All Women*, New York: The Free Press, 2004

Skenazy, L., *Free Range Kids: How to Raise Safe, Self-Reliant Children (Without Going Nuts with Worry)*, San Francisco: Jossey Bass, 2010

Williams, F., *Breasts: A Natural and Unnatural History*, New York: W. W. Norton & Company, 2012

Wolf, J. B., *Is Breast Best?: Taking on the Breastfeeding Experts and the New High Stakes of Motherhood*, New York: New York University Press, 2012

Endnotes

Introduction

1 Hirschman, C. and M. Butler (1981) 'Trends and differentials in breast feeding: an update', *Demography*, vol. 18, pp. 39–54.

2 Weaver, L. (2009) *Feeding Babies in the 21st Century: Breast is still best, but for different reasons*, London: History & Policy. Available at: www.historyandpolicy. org/papers/policy-paper-89.html (accessed 18 September 2012).

3 Health and Social Care Information Centre and IFF Research (2012) *Infant Feeding Survey 2010: Summary*, Leeds: Health and Social Care Information Centre, pp. 4–5. Available at: catalogue.ic.nhs.uk/publications/public-health/ surveys/infant-feed-surv-2010/ifs-uk-2010-sum.pdf (accessed 27 October 2013).

4 Centers for Disease Control and Prevention (2013) *Breastfeeding Report Card: United States 2013*, Atlanta: Centers for Disease Control and Prevention. Available at: www.cdc.gov/breastfeeding/pdf/2013BreastfeedingReportCard.pdf.

5 Australian Institute of Health and Welfare (2012) *Australia's Health 2012*, Canberra: Australian Institute of Health and Welfare. Available at: www.aihw.gov. au/publication-detail/?id=10737422172&tab=3 (accessed 14 November 2013).

6 Lawrence Garter, a paediatrician and the chair of the Breastfeeding Section of the American Association of Pediatricians, told *Newsweek* in 1997, 'It's hard to come out and say, "Your baby is going to be stupider or sicker if you don't breastfeed." But that's what the literature says.' It doesn't, actually, Lawrence. But thanks for making millions of women feel so much worse. Nice job. See Glick, D. (1997) 'Rooting for intelligence', *Newsweek*, 3 March, p. 32.

Part 1: The theory

1 Why mothers bottle-feed

1 Boseley, S. (2013) 'Breastfeeding problems rarely lead to serious illness, study shows', *Guardian*, 20 March. Available at: www.theguardian.com/ lifeandstyle/2013/mar/20/breastfeeding-myths-dispelled (accessed 27 November 2013).

2 Email correspondence from Anne Woods, Deputy Director, UK Baby Friendly Initiative, 22 January 2013. The two UNICEF and WHO documents were *Protecting, Promoting and Supporting Breastfeeding* (1989) and *Global Strategy for Infant and Young Child Feeding* (2002).

3 Neifert, M. et al. (1990) 'The influence of breast surgery, breast appearance, and pregnancy-induced breast changes on lactation sufficiency as measured by infant weight gain', *Birth*, vol. 17, no. 1, pp. 31–8.

4 Odom, E. C., R. Li, K. S. Scanlon, C. G. Perrine and L. Grummer-Strawn (2013) 'Reasons for earlier than desired cessation of breastfeeding', *Pediatrics*, vol. 131, no. 3, pp. e726–32, doi: 10.1542/peds.2012–1295.

Hinsliff-Smith, K., R. Spencer and D. Walsh (2013) 'Realities, difficulties, and outcomes for mothers choosing to breastfeed: primigravid mothers' experience in the early postpartum period (6–8 weeks)', *Midwifery*, published online 9 October doi: 10.1016/j.midw.2013.10.001.

Huggins, K. E., E. S. Petok and O. Mireles (2000) 'Markers of lactation insufficiency: a study of 34 mothers', *Issues in Clinical Lactation*, pp. 25–35.

Cannon, A., H. Jacobson and B. Morgan (n.d.) *Living with Chronic Low Milk Supply: A Basic Guide*, MOBI Motherhood International. Available at: www.mobimotherhood.org/low-milk-supply.

5   Cassar-Uhl, D. (2009) *Supporting Mothers with Mammary Hypoplasia*, La Leche League International. Available at: www.llli.org/llleaderweb/lv/lviss2-3-2009p4.html (accessed 29 November 2013).

6   Heise, A. M. and D. Wiessinger (2011) 'Dysphoric milk ejection reflex: a case report', *International Breastfeeding Journal*, vol. 6, no. 6, doi: 10.1186/1746-4358-6-6.

Brown, A. (2013) 'Maternal trait personality and breastfeeding duration: the importance of confidence and social support', *Journal of Advanced Nursing*, published online, 6 August, doi: 10.1111/jan.12219.

Schmeid, V. and D. Lupton (2001) 'Blurring the boundaries: breastfeeding and maternal subjectivity', *Sociology of Health and Illness*, vol. 23, no. 2, pp. 234–50.

7   Schulmeister, U., I. Swoboda, S. Quirce, B. de la Hoz, M. Ollert, G. Pauli, R. Valenta and S. Spitzauer (2007) 'Sensitization to human milk', *Clinical and Experimental Allergy*, vol. 38, no. 1, pp. 60–8.

8   Office for National Statistics (2013) 'Births in England and Wales, 2012'. Available at: www.ons.gov.uk/ons/rel/vsob1/birth-summary-tables—england-and-wales/2012/stb-births-in-england-and-wales-2012.html (accessed 3 December 2013).

9   Australia Bureau of Statistics (2013) '3301.0 – Births, Australia, 2012'. Available at: www.abs.gov.au/ausstats/abs@.nsf/mf/3301.0 (accessed 3 December 2013).

10 WebMD, 'Erectile dysfunction health centre'. Available at: www.webmd.com/erectile-dysfunction/guide/erectile-dysfunction-basics (accessed 3 December 2013).

11 Davis, L. S. (2013) 'Is the medical community failing breast-feeding moms?' *Time*, 7 January. Available at: http://edition.cnn.com/2013/01/03/health/medical-breastfeeding/ (accessed 3 December 2013).

12 Neifert, M. (2011) 'Prevention of breastfeeding tragedies', P

13 Nommsen-Rivers, L. A., C. J. Chantry, J. M. Peerson, R. J. Cohen and K. G. Dewey (2010) 'Delayed onset of lactogenesis among first-time mothers is related to maternal obesity and factors associated with ineffective breastfeeding', *American Journal of Clinical Nutrition*, vol. 92, no. 3, pp. 574–84.

14 Wagner, E. A., C. J. Chantry, K. G. Dewey and L. A. Nommsen-Rivers (2013) 'Breastfeeding concerns at 3 and 7 days postpartum and feeding status at 2 months', *Pediatrics*, published online, 23 September, doi: 10.1542/peds.2013-0724.

15 Odom, E. C. et al. (2013).

16 Stuebe, A. (2012) 'How often does breastfeeding just not work?' *Breastfeeding Medicine*, 15 October. Available at: bfmed.wordpress.com/2012/10/15/how-often-does-breastfeeding-just-not-work/#comments (accessed 28 November 2012).

17 Matias et al. (2009) *Maternal and Child Nutrition*.

18 Otoo et al. JHL.
19 Stewart-Knox, B., K. Gardiner and M. Wright (2003) 'What is the problem with breast-feeding? A qualitative analysis of infant feeding perceptions', *Journal of Human Nutrition and Dietetics*, vol. 16, no. 4, pp. 265–73.
20 Hausman, B. (2003) *Mother's Milk: Breastfeeding Controversies in American Culture*, New York: Routledge, p. 93.
21 An interesting qualitative study from Australia of lower socio-economic mothers actually found that breastfeeding is considered normative. Sheehan, A., V. Schmied and L. Barclay (2010) 'Complex decisions: theorizing women's infant feeding decisions in the first 6 weeks after birth', *Journal of Advanced Nursing*, vol. 66, no. 2, pp. 371–80.
22 Phone interview with Dr Brooke Scelza, 2 December 2013.
23 'Statutory maternity pay and leave: employer guide'. Available at: www.gov.uk/ employers-maternity-pay-leave/entitlement (accessed 6 December 2013).
24 'Parental leave'. Available at: www.fairwork.gov.au/leave/parental-leave/pages/ default.aspx (accessed 6 December 2013).
25 Skype interview with Dr Katie Hinde, 16 November 2013.
26 Hauck, Y. L. and V. F. Irurita (2002) 'Constructing compatibility: managing breast-feeding and weaning from the mother's perspective', *Qualitative Health Research*, vol. 12, no. 7, pp. 897–914.
27 Dyson, L., F. M. McCormick and M. J. Renfrew (2005) 'Interventions for promoting the initiation of breastfeeding', *Cochrane Database of Systematic Reviews*, issue no. 2, article no. CD001688, doi: 10.1002/14651858.CD001688.pub2.
28 Hoddinott, P., L. C. A. Craig, J. Britten and R. M. McInnes (2012) 'A serial qualitative interview study of infant feeding experiences: idealism meets realism', *BMJ Open*, vol. 2, p. e000504, doi: 10.1136/bmjopen-2011-000504.
29 Kelleher, C. (2006) 'The physical challenges of early breastfeeding', *Social Sciences and Medicine*, vol. 63, pp. 2727–38.
30 Trickey, H. and M. Newhurn (2013) *Infant Feeding Impact Review Summary Report: Methods, Findings and Recommendations*, London: NCT.
31 Skype interview with Dr Katie Hinde, 16 November 2013.
32 Comment by 'Jayne' in response to Lee, K. (2011) 'Do I laugh or cry?', *Breastfeeding Medicine*. Available at: bfmed.wordpress.com/2011/04/29/ do-i-laugh-or-cry/#comment-932 (accessed 11 November 2013).
33 Skype interview with Dr Mandy Belfort, 21 November 2013.
34 Riggins, C., M. B. Rosenman and K. A. Szucs (2012) 'Breastfeeding experiences among physicians', *Breastfeeding Medicine*, vol. 7, no. 3, pp. 151–4, doi: 10.1089/bfm.2011.0045.
35 See, for example, the comments of breastfeeding researcher Dr Sam Oddie about the risk of serious illness for babies who aren't breastfeeding well: 'As far as I'm concerned, the answer isn't more formula-feeding, but better support for breastfeeding from the outset.' Also, comments attributed to Anne Woods, deputy programme manager for UNICEF's Baby Friendly Initiative: the number of babies who could not feed is negligible and only a very small percentage – about 1% – of women would struggle to make enough milk. Also, 'The numbers who breastfeed in this country do not reflect the numbers who could breastfeed if they had effective support.' Both quotes from Boseley, S. (2013) 'Breastfeeding problems rarely lead to serious illness, study shows', *Guardian*, 20 March. Available at: www.theguardian.com/lifeandstyle/2013/mar/20/breastfeeding-myths-dispelled (accessed 27 November 2013).

36 For an excellent and engaging examination of how chemicals affect breasts and the hormonal system, see Williams, F. (2012) *Breasts: A Natural and Unnatural History*, New York: W. W. Norton & Company.

37 Odom, E. C. et al. (2013).

38 Hoddinott, P. et al. (2012).

2 Why bottle-feeding will not make your baby fat, sick or stupid

1 Bolling, K., C. Grant, B. Hamlyn and A. Thornton (2007) *Infant Feeding Survey 2005*, Leeds: Health and Social Care Information Centre.

2 Howie, P., J. S. Forsyth, S. A. Ogston, A. Clark and C. D. Florey (1990) 'Protective effect of breast feeding against infection', *BMJ*, vol. 300, no. 6716, pp. 11–16.

3 Wolf, J. B. (2011) *Is Breast Best? Taking on the Breastfeeding Experts and the New High Stakes of Motherhood*, New York: New York University Press, pp. 24–5.

4 Ip, S. et al. (2007) *Breastfeeding and Maternal and Infant Health Outcomes in Developed Countries*, Evidence Report/Technology Assessment No. 153/AHRQ Publication No. 07-E007, Rockville: Agency for Healthcare Research and Quality (AHRQ).

5 As an example, this study into breastfeeding and mothers' responses to their babies' cry only looked at 17 mother–infant pairs yet was published in a very reputable journal. Kilyoung, K. et al. (2011) 'Breastfeeding, brain activation to own infant cry, and maternal sensitivity', *Journal of Child Psychology and Psychiatry*, vol. 52, no. 8, pp. 907–15.

6 As an example, the American Association of Pediatrics, in the same policy document that calls for infant feeding to be treated as a public health issue, admits: 'Major methodologic issues have been raised as to the quality of some of these studies, especially as to the size of the study populations, quality of the data set, inadequate adjustment for confounders, absence of distinguishing between "any" or "exclusive" breastfeeding, and lack of a defined causal relationship between breastfeeding and the specific outcome.' Yet this is never reflected in any of the body's material encouraging women to breastfeed. See Eidelman, A. and R. Schanler (2012) 'Policy statement: breastfeeding and the use of human milk', *Pediatrics*, vol. 129, no. 3, pp. e827–41. It's also worth pointing out that Dr Eidelman, one of the lead authors of this report, is also the president of the Association of Breastfeeding Medicine. To my mind that's a little like asking the President of the Pineapple Growers' Society to write the definitive policy on whether we should be eating pineapples.

7 Ip, S. et al. (2007), p. vi.

8 Law, J. (2000) 'The politics of breastfeeding: assessing risk, dividing labor', *Signs*, vol. 25, no. 2, pp. 407–50.

9 We have adopted clear, predefined criteria for selecting the research we have reviewed here. Firstly, studies of 'grade A' quality were sought, i.e. meta-analyses and systematic reviews, randomised trials and high-quality observational studies. (The latter were used when other studies were not available.) Secondly, studies were individually examined for quality and bias. Most specifically, we looked for clarity in what was actually being tested, how the test group and comparison group were selected and their demographics, appropriate outcome measures, proper statistical methods and reporting, correct consideration and adjustment for confounding factors and appropriate conclusions and abstract synopsis. Thirdly, high-quality review articles were also included when appropriate.

10 Saint, S. et al. (2000) 'Journal reading habits of internists', *Journal of General Internal Medicine*, vol. 15, p. 883.

11 Quigley, M. A., Y. J. Kelly and A. Sacker (2007) 'Breastfeeding and hospitalization for diarrheal and respiratory infection in the United Kingdom millennium cohort study', *Pediatrics*, vol. 119, no. 4, pp. 837–42.

Ip, S. et al. (2007), pp. 40–1.

Nishimura, T., J. Suzue and H. Kaji (2009) 'Breastfeeding reduces the severity of respiratory syncytial virus infection among young infants: a multi-centre prospective study', *Pediatrics International*, vol. 51, no. 6, pp. 812–16.

Libster, R. et al. (2009) 'Breastfeeding prevents severe disease in full-term infants with acute respiratory infection', *Pediatric Infectious Disease Journal*, vol. 28, no. 2, pp. 131–4.

12 Ip, S. et al. (2007), p. 27.

13 Oddy, W. H. et al. (2003) 'Breast feeding and respiratory morbidity in infancy: a birth cohort study', *Archives of Diseases in Childhood*, vol. 88, pp. 224–8.

14 Cushing, A. et al. (1998) 'Breast feeding reduces risk of respiratory illness in infants', *American Journal of Epidemiology*, vol. 147, no. 9, pp. 863–70.

15 Bachrach, V. R., E. Schwarz and L. R. Bachrach (2003) 'Breastfeeding and the risk of hospitalization for respiratory disease in infancy', *Archives of Pediatrics and Adolescent Medicine*, vol. 157, no. 3, pp. 237–43.

16 Kramer, M. S. et al. (2001) 'Promotion of breastfeeding intervention trial (PROBIT): a randomized trial in the Republic of Belarus', *Journal of the American Medical Association*, vol. 285, pp. 413–20.

17 Ip, S. et al. (2007), p. 27.

18 Ip, S. et al. (2007), p. 27.

Howie, P. et al. (1990), pp. 11–16.

Duffy, L. C. et al. (1997) 'Exclusive breastfeeding protects against bacterial colonization and day care exposure to otitis media', *Pediatrics*, vol. 100, no. 4, pp. e7–15.

Zielhuis, G. A., E. W. Heuvelmans-Heinen, G. H. Rach et al. (1989) 'Environmental risk factors for otitis media with effusion in preschool children', *Scandinavian Journal of Primary Health Care*, vol. 7, pp. 33–8.

19 Duffy, L. C. et al. (1997), e7–15.

20 Lanphear, B. P., R. S. Byrd, P. Auinger and C. B. Hall (1997) 'Increasing prevalence of recurrent otitis media among children in the United States', *Pediatrics*, vol. 99, no. 3, p. e1.

21 Paradise, J. et al. (1997) 'Otitis media in 2253 Pittsburgh-area infants: prevalence and risk factors during the first two years of life', *Pediatrics*, vol. 99, no. 3, pp. 229–30.

22 Ip, S. et al. (2007), pp. 37–8.

Kramer, M. S. et al. (2001), pp. 413–20.

Quigley, M. A., Y. J. Kelly and A. Sacker (2007) 'Breastfeeding and hospitalization for diarrheal and respiratory infection in the United Kingdom millennium cohort study', *Pediatrics*, vol. 119, no. 4, pp. 837–42.

Duffy, L. C. et al. (1997) 'Exclusive breastfeeding protects against bacterial colonization and day care exposure to otitis media', *Pediatrics*, vol. 100, no. 4, pp. e7–15.

Chien, P. F. and P. W. Howie (2001) 'Breast milk and the risk of opportunistic infection in infancy in industrialized and non-industrialized settings', *Advances in Nutritional Research*, vol. 10, pp. 69–104.

23 Kramer, M. et al. (2001), pp. 413–20.

24 Quigley, M. A., P. Cumberland, J. M. Cowden and L. C. Rodrigues (2006) 'How protective is breast feeding against diarrhoeal disease in infants in 1990s England? A case-control study', *Archives of Disease in Childhood*, vol. 91, no. 3, pp. 245–50.

25 Many studies and anecdotal reports show that mothers are not taught how to safely prepare bottles. One systematic review, which looked at more than 13,000 mothers, found: 'Mothers reported receiving little information on bottle-feeding . . . Mistakes in preparation of bottle-feeds were common.' The authors argued that 'Inadequate information and support for mothers who decide to bottle-feed may put the health of their babies at risk.' Lakshman, R., D. Ogilvie and K. K. Ong (2009) 'Mothers' experiences of bottle-feeding: a systematic review of qualitative and quantitative studies', *Archives of Disease in Childhood*, vol. 94, pp. 596–601.

26 Hascoet, J. M. et al. (2011) 'Effect of formula composition on the development of infant gut microbiota', *Journal of Pediatric Gastroenterology and Nutrition*, vol. 52, no. 6, pp. 756–62.

27 Victora, C. G. et al. (2003) 'Anthropometry and body composition of 18 year old men according to duration of breast feeding: birth cohort study from Brazil', *BMJ*, vol. 327, p. 904.

Kwok, M. K. et al. (2009) 'Does breastfeeding in childhood protect against childhood overweight? Hong Kong's "Children of 1997" birth cohort', *International Journal of Epidemiology*, electronic publication, vol. 38, no. 1, pp. 1–9.

Al-Qaoud, N. and P. Prakash (2009) 'Can breastfeeding and its duration determine the overweight status of Kuwaiti children at the age of 3–6 years?', *European Journal of Clinical Medicine*, vol. 63, no. 8, pp. 1041–3.

Kramer, M. S. et al. (2007) 'Effects of prolonged and exclusive breastfeeding on child height, weight, adiposity, and blood pressure at age 6.5y: evidence from a large randomized trial', *American Journal of Clinical Nutrition*, vol. 86, no. 6, pp. 1717–21.

Li, L., T. J. Parson and C. Power (2003) 'Breast feeding and obesity in childhood: cross sectional study', *BMJ*, vol. 327, no. 420, pp. 904–5.

Parsons, T. J., C. Power and O. Manor (2003) 'Infant feeding and obesity through the life course', *Archives of Disease in Childhood*, vol. 88, no. 9, pp. 793–4.

28 Fewtrell, M. S. (2004) 'The longterm benefits of having been breastfed', *Current Pediatrics*, vol. 14, pp. 97–103.

Gillman, M. W. et al. (2001) 'Risk of overweight among adults who are breastfed as infants', *JAMA*, vol. 285, pp. 2461–7.

Bergman, K. E. et al. (2003) 'Early determinants of childhood overweight and adiposity in a birth cohort study: role of breast feeding', *International Journal of Obesity*, vol. 27, p. 162.

Arenz, S. et al. (2004) 'Breastfeeding and childhood obesity: a systematic review', *International Journal of Obesity Related Metabolic Disorders*, vol. 28, no. 10, pp. 1247–56.

Harder, T. et al. (2005) 'Duration of breastfeeding and risk of overweight: a meta-analysis', *American Journal of Epidemiology*, vol. 162, no. 5, pp. 397–403.

Owen, C. G. et al. (2005) 'Effect of infant feeding on the risk of obesity across the life course: a quantitative review of published evidence', *Pediatrics*, vol. 115, no. 5, pp. 1367–77.

29 Ip, S. et al. (2007), p. 65.
30 Beyerlein, A. and R. von Kries (2011) 'Breastfeeding and body composition in children: will there ever be conclusive empirical evidence for a protective effect against overweight?', *American Journal of Clinical Nutrition*, vol. 94, no. 6 (suppl.), pp. 1772S–75.
31 Horta, B. and C. Victora (2013) *Long-term Effects of Breastfeeding: A Systematic Review*, Geneva: World Health Organization, p. 16.
32 Robinson, S. et al. (2013) 'Type of milk feeding in infancy and health behaviours in adult life: findings from the Hertfordshire cohort study', *British Journal of Nutrition*, vol. 109, no. 6, pp. 1114–22.
33 Heinig, M. J., L. A. Nommsen, J. M. Peerson et al. (1993) 'Energy and protein intakes of breast-fed and formula-fed infants during the first year of life and their association with growth velocity: the DARLING study', *American Journal of Clinical Nutrition*, vol. 58, pp. 152–61.
34 Hunsberger, M. et al. (2012) 'Infant feeding practices and prevalence of obesity in eight European countries – the IDEFICS study', *Public Health Nutrition*, published online, 24 August, doi: 10.1017/S1368980012003850.
35 Heinig, M. J., L. A. Nommsen, J. M. Peerson et al. (1993).
36 Li, R., J. Magadia, S. B. Fein and L. M. Grummer-Strawn (2012) 'Risk of bottle-feeding for rapid weight gain during the first year of life', *Archives of Pediatric and Adolescent Medicine*, vol. 166, no. 5, pp. 431–6.
37 Heinig, M. J., L. A. Nommsen, J. M. Peerson et al. (1993).
38 Ventura, A. K., G. K. Beauchamp and J. A. Mennella (2012) 'Infant regulation of intake: the effect of free glutamate content in infant formulas', *American Journal of Clinical Nutrition*, vol. 95, no. 4, pp. 875–81.
39 Hediger, M. L., M. F. Overpeck, R. J. Kuczmarski and W. J. Ruan (2001) 'Association between infant breastfeeding and overweight in young children' *JAMA*, vol. 285, no. 19, pp. 2453–60.
    Al-Qaoud, N. and P. Prakash (2009).
40 Ip, S. et al. (2007), p. 78.
41 Sadauskaite-Kuehne, V. et al. (2004) 'Longer breastfeeding is an independent protective factor against development of type 1 diabetes mellitus in childhood', *Diabetes/Metabolism Research and Reviews*, vol. 20, no. 2, pp. 150–7.
42 Bodington, M. J., P. G. McNally and A. C. Burden (1994) 'Cow's milk and type 1 childhood diabetes: no increase risk', *Diabetic Medicine*, vol. 11, no. 7, pp. 663–5.
    Couper, J. J. et al. (1999) 'Lack of association between duration of breast-feeding or introduction of cow's milk and development of islet autoimmunity', *Diabetes*, vol. 48, no. 11, pp. 2145–9.
43 Hummel, M., M. Fuchtenbusch, M. Schenker and A. G. Ziegler (2000) 'No major association of breast-feeding, vaccinations and childhood viral diseases with early islet autoimmunity in the German BABYDIAB study', *Diabetes Care*, vol. 23, no. 7, pp. 969–74.
44 Davis, J. N. et al. (2007) 'Influence of breastfeeding on obesity and type 2 diabetes risk factors in Latino youth with a family history of type 2 diabetes', *Diabetes Care*, vol. 30, no. 4.
    Evenhouse, E. and S. Reilly (2005) 'Improving estimates of the benefits of breastfeeding using sibling comparisons to reduce selection bias', *Health Services Research*, vol. 40, no. 6, part 1, pp. 1781–802.
45 Mayer-Davis, E. J. et al. (2008) 'Breastfeeding and type 2 diabetes in the youth of three ethnic groups', *Diabetes Care*, vol. 31, no. 3, pp. 470–5.

46 Caspi, A. et al. (2007) 'Moderation of breastfeeding effects on the IQ by genetic variation in fatty acid metabolism', *Proceedings of the National Academy of Sciences*, vol. 104, no. 47, pp. 18860–5.

47 Bartels, M., C. E. M. van Beijsterveldt and D. I. Boomsma (2009) 'Breastfeeding, maternal education and cognitive function: a prospective study in twins', *Behavior Genetics*, vol. 39, pp. 616–22.

Rees, D. I. and J. A. Sabia (2009) 'The effect of breast feeding on education attainment: evidence from sibling data', *Journal of Human Capital*, vol. 3, no. 1, pp. 43–72.

Kramer, M. S. et al. (2008) 'Breastfeeding and cognitive development: new evidence from a large randomised trial', *Archives of General Psychiatry*, vol. 65, no. 5, pp. 578–84.

48 Ip, S. et al. (2007), p. 53.

49 Drover, J. R. et al. (2009) 'Three randomized controlled trials of early long-chain polyunsaturated fatty acid supplementation on mean-end problem solving in nine-month olds', *Child Development*, vol. 80, no. 5, pp. 1376–84.

50 Cornucopia Institute (n.d.) *Questions and Answers About DHA/AHA and Infant Formula*, Cornucopia, Wisconsin: Cornucopia Institute. Available at: cornucopia.org/DHA/DHA_QuestionsAnswers.pdf (accessed 26 November 2013).

51 For example, this study by Agostini found a similar level of infant development between supplemented formula-fed and breastfed infants: Agostini, C. (2008) 'Role of long-chain polyunsaturated fatty acids in the first year of life', *Journal of Pediatric Gastroenterology and Nutrition*, vol. 47, suppl. 2, pp. S41–4.

52 Delgado-Noguera, M. F., J. A. Calvache and X. Bonfill Cosp (2010) 'Supplementation with long chain polyunsaturated fatty acids (LCPUFA) to breastfeeding mothers for improving child growth and development', *Cochrane Database of Systematic Reviews 2010*, no. 12., article no. CD007901, doi: 10.1002/14651858.CD007901.pub2.

53 Colombo, J., S. E. Carlson, C. L. Cheatham, D. J. Shaddy, E. H. Kerling, J. M. Thodosoff, K. M. Gustafson and C. Brez (2013) 'Long-term effects of LCPUFA supplementation on childhood cognitive outcomes', *American Journal of Clinical Nutrition*, vol. 98, no. 2, pp. 403–12.

54 Caspi, A. et al. (2007) 'Moderation of breastfeeding effects on the IQ by genetic variation in fatty acid metabolism', *Proceedings of the National Academy of Sciences*, vol. 104, no. 47, pp. 18860–5. This particular study demonstrated that breastfed children who have a gene variant that is involved in the production of the main LCPUFAs present in human breast milk have lower IQs, i.e. they are not able to benefit from the positive effect of the LCPUFAs in the breast milk and have IQs similar to those they would have had they been fed standard formula.

55 FAQs on Bellamy's Organic website. Available at: bellamysorganic.com.au/faqs/#dha_ara (accessed 26 November 2013).

56 Der, G., G. D. Batty and I. J. Deary (2006) 'Effect of breast feeding on intelligence in children: prospective study, sibling pairs analysis, and meta-analysis', *British Medical Journal*, vol. 333, pp. 945–8.

57 Jacobson, S. W., L. M. Chiodo and J. L. Jacobson (1999) 'Breastfeeding effects on intelligence quotient in 4- and 11-year-old children', *Pediatrics*, vol. 103, no. 5, p. e71. The authors put it very nicely in their summary of findings: 'The mother's decision to breastfeed, particularly for an extended period, presumably reflects her concern with her infant's welfare and her motivation and ability to stimulate

and enrich her child's development, which are at least partially independent of social class and education.'

58 Horta, B. and C. Victora (2013) *Long-term Effects of Breastfeeding: A Systematic Review*, Geneva: World Health Organization, p. 61.

59 Kramer, M. S. et al. (2008).

60 Kramer, M. S. et al. (2008).

61 Lavelli, M. and M. Poli (1998) 'Early mother-infant interaction during breast- and bottle-feeding', *Infant Behavior and Development*, vol. 21, pp. 667–84.

62 Kramer, M. S. et al. (2008).

63 Tamis-LeMonda, C., J. D. Shannon, N. J. Cabrera and M. E. Lamb (2004) 'Fathers and mothers at play with their 2- and 3-year olds: contributions to language and cognitive development', *Child Development*, vol. 75, no. 6, pp. 1806–20. Please note that we are not suggesting that father–child play has the same potential impact on babies' IQ as breastfeeding; however, if fathers are more involved with babies, for example through bottle-feeding, that is linked with positive childhood development.

64 Medina, J. (2010) *Brain Rules for Babies*, Seattle: Pear Press, p. 129.

65 Dr Medina also urged mothers to breastfeed, though he doesn't critically analyse the research and references only three studies, one of which finds no association between breastfeeding and intelligence. Medina, J. (2010), pp. 126–42.

66 Belfort, M. B. et al. (2013) 'Infant feeding and childhood cognition at ages 3 and 7 years: effects of breastfeeding duration and exclusivity', *JAMA Pediatrics*, vol. 167, no. 9, pp. 836–44, doi: 10.1001/jamapediatrics.2013.455.

67 Skype interview with Dr Mandy Belfort, 21 November 2013.

68 Murkoff, H. and H. Mazel (2009) *What to Expect When You're Expecting* (4th edition), London: Simon and Schuster, p. 330.

69 Klaus, M. et al. (1972) 'Maternal attachment: importance of the first postpartum days', *New England Journal of Medicine*, vol. 286, no. 9, pp. 460–3.

70 As detailed in Eyer, D. (1992) *Mother-Infant Bonding: A Scientific Fiction*, New Haven: Yale University Press. See, for example, Lamb, M. (1982) 'Early contact and maternal-infant bonding: one decade later', *Pediatrics*, vol. 70, no. 5, pp. 763–8.

71 Corsini, R. J. (1999) *The Dictionary of Psychology*, Philadelphia: Brunner/Mazel, p. 123 defines 'bonding' as being two-way, whereas Klaus and Kennell refer to the bond of the mother to the child. See Kennell, J. and M. Klaus (1998) 'Bonding: recent observations that alter perinatal care', *Pediatrics in Review*, vol. 19, pp. 4–12.

72 Bowlby, J. (1958) 'The nature of the child's tie to his mother', *International Journal of Psychoanalysis*, vol. 39, pp. 350–73.

73 Britton, J. R., H. L. Britton and V. Gronwaldt (2006) 'Breastfeeding, sensitivity and attachment', *Pediatrics*, vol. 118, no. 5, pp. e1436–43.

74 Else-Quest, N., J. Hyde and R. Clark (2003) 'Breastfeeding, bonding and the mother-infant relationship', *Merrill-Palmer Quarterly*, vol. 49, no. 4, pp. 495–517.

75 Else-Quest, N., J. Hyde and R. Clark (2003).

76 Jansen, J., C. de Weerth and M. Riksen-Walraven (2008) 'Breastfeeding and the mother-infant relationship: a review', *Developmental Review*, vol. 28, pp. 503–21.

77 Kosfeld, M. et al. (2005) 'Oxytocin increases trust in humans', *Nature*, vol. 435, pp. 673–6.

78 Uvnas-Moberg, K. (1998) 'Oxytocin may mediate the benefits of positive social interaction and emotions', *Psychoneuroendocrinology*, vol. 23, no. 8, pp. 819–35.

79 Perry, B. D. (2001) *Bonding and Attachment in Maltreated Children*, Houston: Child Trauma Academy. Available at: aia.berkeley.edu/strengthening_connections/handouts/perry/Bonding%20and%20Attachment.pdf (accessed 27 November 2013).

80 Feldman, R. (2007) 'Parent-infant synchrony: biological foundations and developmental outcomes', *Current Directions in Psychological Science*, vol. 16, pp. 340–5.

81 Ip, S. et al. (2007), p. 112.

82 Palumbo, P. (2009) 'Breastfeed and say bye bye to baby weight: does breastfeeding really speed weight loss?', *Momma Data*, 13 November. Available at: mommadata.blogspot.com.au/2009/11/breastfeed-and-say-bye-bye-to-baby.html (accessed 19 November 13).

83 Flaherman, V. J., J. Aby, A. E. Burgos, K. A. Lee, M. D. Cabana and T. B. Newman (2013) 'Effect of early limited formula on duration and exclusivity of breastfeeding in at-risk infants: an RCT', *Pediatrics*, published online, 13 May 2013, doi: 10.1542/peds.2012-2809.

84 Nommsen-Rivers, L. A., C. J. Chantry, J. M. Peerson, R. J. Cohen and K. G. Dewey (2010) 'Delayed onset of lactogenesis among first-time mothers is related to maternal obesity and factors associated with ineffective breastfeeding', *American Journal of Clinical Nutrition*, vol. 92, no. 3, pp. 574–84.

85 Williams, F. (2012), *Breasts: A Natural and Unnatural History*, New York: W. W. Norton & Co., p. 198.

86 Williams, F. (2012), p. 209.

87 Rippenyoung, P. and M. Noonan (2012) 'Is breastfeeding truly cost free? Income consequences of breastfeeding for women', *American Sociological Review*, vol. 77, no. 2, pp. 244–67.

88 Skype interview with Dr Mandy Belfort, 21 November 2013.

89 The Economist (2013) 'Trouble at the lab', *The Economist*, 19–25 October, pp. 22–3.

90 The most famous of these is a sting by the editor of the prestigious *British Medical Journal*, Fiona Godlee. She sent an article containing eight deliberate errors in study design, analysis and interpretation to 200 of the journal's regular reviewers. On average, the reviewers found only two of the errors. Some found none at all. (Godlee, F., C. R. Gale and C. N. Martyn (1998) 'Effect on the quality of peer review of blinding reviewers and asking them to sign their reports: a randomised controlled trial', *JAMA*, vol. 280, pp. 237–40.) Another, more controversial, paper argues: 'most research findings are false'. (Ioannidis, J. P. A. (2005) 'Why most published research findings are false', *PLoS Med*, vol. 2, no. 8, pp. e124, doi: 10.1371/journal.pmed.0020124.)

91 The prestigious journal *Nature* introduced a new checklist for researchers in 2013 that it hopes will improve the quality of research submitted and published. The American government's health research agency, the National Institutes of Health, is also looking at ways to reduce what one of its officials called 'an epidemic of unreproducible results'. See Butterworth, T. (2013) 'Taxpayer-funded journal walks back BPA cancer claim after statistical meltdown', *Forbes*, 26 September. Available at: www.forbes.com/sites/trevorbutterworth/2013/09/26/taxpayer-

funded-journal-walks-back-bpa-cancer-claim-after-statistical-meltdown/?utm_so
urce=alertscalledoutcomment&utm_medium=email&utm_campaign=20131002
(accessed 7 January 2014).
92 Stanley, S. (n.d.) 'The breastfeeding police', *Parenting.com*. Available at: www.
parenting.com/article/the-breastfeeding-police (accessed 24 October 2013).
93 Bottle Babies. Available at: www.bottlebabies.org (accessed 26 November 2013).

3 The Breastfeeding Echo Chamber: how everything you read reinforces 'breast is best'

1   He's obviously not really called Joe. This conversation did happen, though.
2   Stevens, E. E., T. E. Patrick and R. Pickler (2009) 'A history of infant feeding',
Journal of Perinatal Education, vol. 8, no. 2, pp. 32–9.
3   Stevens, E. E. et al. (2009).
4   Stevens, E. E. et al. (2009).
5   Blum, L. (1999), *At the Breast. Ideologies of Breastfeeding and Motherhood in
the Contemporary United States*. Boston: Beacon, p. 22.
6   Wolf, J. B. (2011) *Is Breast Best? Taking on the Breastfeeding Experts and the New
High Stakes of Motherhood*, New York: New York University Press, p. 1.
7   Stevens, E. E. et al. (2009).
8   Stevens, E. E. et al. (2009).
9   Wolf, J. B. (2011), p. 3.
10 Blum, L. (1999), p. 31.
11 Weaver, L. (2009) *Feeding Babies in the 21st Century: Breast is still best, but for
different reasons*, London: History & Policy. Available at: www.historyandpolicy.
org/papers/policy-paper-89.html (accessed 18 September 2012).
12 Hirschman, C. and M. Butler (1981) 'Trends and differentials in breast feeding: an
update', *Demography*, vol. 18, pp. 39–54.
13 La Leche League (2012) 'La Leche League philosophy'. Available at: www.llli.org/
philosophy.html?m=1,0,1 (accessed 5 November 2013).
14 La Leche League (2003) 'A brief history of La Leche League International'.
Available at: www.llli.org/lllihistory.html (accessed 5 November 2013).
15 These studies often accounted for few of the confounding variables we talked
about in Chapter 1, of course.
16 See www.unwater.org/statistics (accessed 13 November 2013).
17 You, D., P. Bastian, J. Wu and T. Wardlaw (2013) *Levels and Trends in Child
Mortality*, New York: UN Inter-agency Group for Child Mortality Estimation.
Available at: www.who.int/maternal_child_adolescent/documents/levels_trends_
child_mortality_2013.pdf (accessed 26 January 2014).
18 UNICEF (2014) 'Infant and young child feeding'. Available at: www.unicef.org/
nutrition/index_breastfeeding.html (accessed 1 November 2013).
19 UNICEF (2012) 'HIV and infant feeding'. Available at: www.unicef.org/nutrition/
index_24827.html (accessed 13 November 2013).
20 WHO (2013) *Global Update on HIV Treatment 2013: Results, Impact and
Opportunities*, Geneva: World Health Organization (WHO). Available at:
www.who.int/hiv/pub/progressreports/update2013/en/index.html (accessed
13 November 2013).
21 Bandyopadhyay, M. (2009) 'Impact of ritual pollution on lactation and
breastfeeding practices in rural West Bengal, India', *International Breastfeeding
Journal*, vol. 4, p. 2, doi: 10.1186/1746-4358-4-2.

22 IRIN (2009) 'Liberia: breaking breastfeeding myths', *IRIN*, 27 November. Available at: www.irinnews.org/report/87226/liberia-breaking-breastfeeding-myths (accessed 13 November 2013).
23 UNICEF (1990) 'Innocenti declaration'. Available at: www.unicef.org/programme/breastfeeding/innocenti.htm (accessed 5 November 2013).
24 Williams, Z. (2013) 'Baby health crisis in Indonesia as formula companies push products', *Guardian*, 15 February. Available at: www.theguardian.com/world/2013/feb/15/babies-health-formula-indonesia-breastfeeding.
25 Newman, M. (2013) '"If you think your baby isn't getting enough, call us . . .": alarmist marketing for Danone formula milk', *Bureau of Investigative Journalism*, 28 June. Available at: www.thebureauinvestigates.com/2013/06/28/if-you-think-your-baby-isnt-getting-enough-call-us-alarmist-marketing-for-danone-formula-milk/ (accessed 13 November 2013).
26 Danone (2012) *Bringing Health through Food to as Many People as Possible: Danone Economic and Social Report 11*, Paris: Danone. Available at: www.danone.ch/danone-media/docs/pdfs/Annual_Report_2011_englisch.pdf p 18. (accessed 14 November 2013).
27 The UNICEF documentary 'Formula for disaster' is available at: www.youtube.com/watch?v=3PBtb-UDhEc (accessed 16 November 2013).
28 Reuters (2013) 'Japan's Meiji to pull out of China's baby formula market', *Reuters*, 25 October. Available at: www.reuters.com/article/2013/10/25/us-china-milk-meiji-idUSBRE99O03L20131025.
29 Suzanne Barston's 'Fearless Formula Feeder' blog. Available at: fearlessformulafeeder.com (accessed 26 November 2013).
30 UBIC Consulting (2010) *Ingredients for the World Infant Formula Market*, Newport Beach: UBIC Consulting. Available at: www.ubic-consulting.com.
31 IRIN (2013) 'Analysis: concern mounts over infant formula additives', *IRIN*, 25 January. Available at: www.irinnews.org/report/97334/analysis-concern-mounts-over-infant-formula-additives (accessed 12 November 2013).
32 UNICEF (2013) 'Breastfeeding is the cheapest and most effective life-saver in history'. Available at: www.unicef.org/media/media_70044.html (accessed 13 November 2013).
33 UBIC Consulting (2010).
34 International Board of Lactation Consultant Examiners (n.d.) 'IBLCE exam facts & figures'. Available at: http://iblce.org/about-iblce/iblce-exam-facts-figures/ (accessed 15 November 2013).
35 For example, the 'Holistic IBCLC' charges 175 euros for a two-hour consultation by Skype. See http://holisticibclc.blogspot.com.au/2011/08/western-mythology-cultivated-by-breast.html (accessed 15 November 2013).
36 Wolf, J. B. (2011), p. 40.
37 Fox, M., C. Berzuini and L. A. Knapp (2013) 'Maternal breastfeeding history and Alzheimer's disease risk', *Journal of Alzheimer's Disease*, uncorrected proof from publisher.
38 Hope, J. (2013) 'Mothers who breastfeed slash their risk of developing Alzheimer's by TWO-THIRDS, claims study', *Daily Mail*, 5 August. Available at: www.dailymail.co.uk/health/article-2384955/Mothers-breastfeed-slash-risk-developing-Alzheimer-s-TWO-THIRDS-claims-study.html (accessed 15 November 2013).
39 JAD (2013) 'Breastfeeding may reduce Alzheimer's risk', *Journal of Alzheimer's Disease* (JAD), 5 August. Available at: www.j-alz.com/node/306 (accessed 15 November 2013).

40 Pearson, C. (2013) 'Breastfeeding may slash Alzheimer's risk, study finds', *Huffington Post*, 6 August. Available at: www.huffingtonpost.com/2013/08/06/breastfeeding-alzheimers_n_3713643.html (accessed 15 November 2013).

41 Heyes, J. D. (2013) 'Breastfeeding proven to lower risk of Alzheimer's in moms', *Natural News*, 9 August. Available at: www.naturalnews.com/041555_alzheimers_breastfeeding_reduced_risk.html (accessed 15 November 2013).

42 NHS Choices (2013) 'Does breastfeeding lower Alzheimer's risk?' Available at: www.nhs.uk/news/2013/08august/pages/does-breastfeeding-lower-alzheimers-risk.aspx (accessed 18 November 2013).

43 Alzheimer's Society (2013) 'Demography'. Available at: www.alzheimers.org.uk/site/scripts/documents_info.php?documentID=412 (accessed 18 November 2013).

44 Narayanan, A. (2012) 'Formula-fed babies don't always overeat: study', *Reuters*, 30 March. Available at: www.reuters.com/article/2012/03/30/us-formula-fed-babies-idUSBRE82T1BA20120330 (accessed 19 November 2013).

45 Wolf, J. B. (2011), p. 39.

46 Kleinman, Z. (2013) 'When breast is not necessarily best: huge pressure is put on today's mothers to breastfeed their babies. One woman's haunting tale reveals how it can lead to great anguish', *Daily Mail*, 19 February. Available at: www.dailymail.co.uk/femail/article-2281396/When-breast-necessarily-best-One-womans-haunting-tale-reveals-lead-great-anguish.html (accessed 19 November 2013).

47 Rosin, H. (2009) 'The case against breast-feeding', *The Atlantic*, 1 April. Available at: www.theatlantic.com/magazine/archive/2009/04/the-case-against-breast-feeding/307311/.

48 Krugman, S., P. Law, D. Fergusson and L. J. Horwood (1999) 'Breastfeeding and IQ', *Pediatrics*, vol. 103, pp. 193–4.

49 Lagan, B. M., M. Sinclair and W. G. Kernohan (2010) 'Internet use in pregnancy informs women's decision making: a web-based survey', *Birth*, vol. 37, no. 2, pp. 106–15.

50 This is another breastfeeding theory designed to scare parents into breastfeeding. It is put about by some breastfeeding advocates that just one bottle of formula will destroy a baby's 'virgin' gut flora and expose her to all sorts of pathogens that she will never recover from, causing a lifetime of allergies. It should be noted that: a) the jury is still very much out on the relationship between allergies and breastfeeding; and b) not one single piece of scientific research has ever looked into 'the virgin gut'. While breastfed babies do have lower incidences of diarrhoea due to the active immune properties of breastfeeding, and these immune properties help to build healthy gut flora, formula-feeding does not 'ruin' anyone's gut, except perhaps that of extreme lactivists who get stomach ulcers over this sort of stuff.

51 Dornan, B. A. and M. H. Oermann (2006) 'Evaluation of breastfeeding web sites for patient education', *MCN American Journal of Maternal Child Nursing*, vol. 31, no. 1, pp. 18–23.

52 NHS Choices (2012) 'Bottle feeding advice'. Available at: www.nhs.uk/conditions/pregnancy-and-baby/pages/bottle-feeding-advice.aspx#close (accessed 21 November 2013).

53 Pregnancy, Birth & Baby (2013) 'Bottle feeding with formula'. Available at: www.pregnancybirthbaby.org.au/bottle-feeding-formula?utm_source=google&utm_medium=cpc&utm_term=formula%20feeding&utm_campaign=Baby+Topics+%28B%29 (accessed 20 November 2013).

54 Telephone interview with Lisa Watson, 20 November 2013.

55 Sydney Morning Herald (2013) 'Feeding frenzy', *Sydney Morning Herald*, 16 February. Available at: www.smh.com.au/lifestyle/feeding-frenzy-20130211-2e793.html#ixzz2lPmj5Bd1 (accessed 23 November 2013).

56 Skype interview with Suzanne Barston, 22 November 2013.

57 Bialik, M. (2011) 'Is this extreme parenting?', *Kveller*, 23 February. Available at: www.kveller.com/blog/parenting/is-this-extreme-parenting/ (accessed 21 November 2013).

58 KellyMom (2011) 'Frequently asked questions about weaning', 28 July. Available at: kellymom.com/ages/weaning/wean-how/weaning_faqs/ (accessed 21 November 2013).

59 'Intensive mothering' is an idea put forward by sociologist Sharon Hays in her influential book *The Cultural Contradictions of Motherhood*. 'Total motherhood' is described by gender studies professor Joan B. Wolf in *Is Breast Best?* and 'the new momism' by Susan J. Douglas in *The Mommy Myth* (see Resources section for full details).

60 Phone interview with Lisa Watson, 23 November 2013.

61 Skype interview with Charlotte Faircloth, 21 November 2013.

62 Skype interview with Suzanne Barston, 22 November 2013.

63 Grumet, J. L. (2012) 'What breastfeeding advocates need to stop saying', *BlogHer*, 4 April. Available at: www.blogher.com/what-breastfeeding-advocates-need-stop-saying (accessed 23 November 2013).

64 Belkin, L. (2013) 'I support you: the conversation we should be having about breastfeeding and formula', *Huffington Post*, 1 August. Available at: www.huffingtonpost.com/2013/08/01/i-support-you-breastfeeding-_n_3685881.html (accessed 23 November 2013).

65 Turner, B. (2013) '10 reasons why breastfeeding is out of fashion', *Telegraph*, 24 June. Available at: www.telegraph.co.uk/women/mother-tongue/10139435/10-reasons-why-breastfeeding-is-out-of-fashion.html (accessed 23 November 2013).

66 Gruttadaro, A. (2013) 'Kim Kardashian Loves Breastfeeding Baby Daughter', *Hollywood Life*, 23 June. Available at: www.hollywoodlife.com/2013/06/23/kim-kardashian-breastfeeding-baby-daughter-kanye-west/ (accessed 23 November 2013).

67 Hilton, P. (2013) 'Kim Kardashian is a lean, mean, breastfeeding machine!', *Perezhilton.com*, 23 June. Available at: perezhilton.com/perezitos/2013-06-23-kim-kardashian-breastfeeding-love-for-baby-north-great-mother (accessed 23 November 2013).

68 The Hollywood Gossip (2013) 'Kim Kardashian: breastfeeding North West like crazy!', 23 June. Available at: www.thehollywoodgossip.com/2013/06/kim-kardashian-breastfeeding-north-west-like-crazy/ (accessed 23 November 2013).

69 Douglas, S. and M. Michaels (2004) *The Mommy Myth: The Idealization of Motherhood and How It Has Undermined All Women*, New York: The Free Press, pp. 110–39.

70 Douglas, S. and M. Michaels (2004), p. 116.

71 This was how Victoria Beckham explained her decision to breastfeed daughter Harper, when she had bottle-fed her three sons: 'I'm doing everything differently this time. I want it all to be natural and perfect for my little girl.' Hilton, P. (2011) 'Victoria Beckham is breastfeeding her first daughter', *Perezhilton.com*, 21 July. Available at: perezhilton.com/fitperez/2011-07-21-victoria-beckham-breastfeeding-daughter#sthash.XF7POOe4.dpbs (accessed 25 November 2013).

72 Douglas, S. and M. Michaels (2004), p. 119.
73 McGinnis, S. (2008) 'The miseducation of Jennifer Lopez', *Baby Center*, 26 March. Available at: blogs.babycenter.com/celebrities/the-miseducation-of-jennifer-lopez/ (accessed 25 November 2013).
74 Daily Mail (n.d.) 'Charities call for baby milk ads ban as Jordan feature "breaks rules"', *Daily Mail*. Available at: www.dailymail.co.uk/health/article-473695/Charities-baby-milk-ads-ban-Jordan-feature-breaks-rules.html (accessed 25 November 2013).
75 Powley, K. (2012) 'Piri Weepu's baby bottle advert ban', *New Zealand Herald*, 5 February. Available at: www.nzherald.co.nz/nz/news/article.cfm?c_id=1&objectid=10783518 (accessed 25 November 2012).
76 Powley, K. (2012) 'Piri Weepu reveals worries for baby's health', *New Zealand Herald*, 12 August. Available at: www.nzherald.co.nz/nz/news/article.cfm?c_id=1&objectid=10826271 (accessed 25 November 2013).
77 TVNZ (2012) 'Close up: Piri Weepu images spark concern over breastfeeding', *ONE News*, 6 February. Available at: tvnz.co.nz/close-up/piri-weepu-images-spark-concern-over-breastfeeding-video-4712946 (accessed 25 November 2012).

4 Guilt, pressure and support

1 Lee, E. (2007) 'Health, morality and infant feeding: British mothers' experience of formula milk use in the early weeks', *Sociology of Health and Illness*, vol. 29, no. 7, pp. 1075–90.
2 Discussion on www.facebook.com/bottlebabies on 18 December 2013 (accessed 18 December 2013).
3 As found in Sheehan, A., V. Schmied and L. Barclay (2010) 'Complex decisions: theorizing women's infant feeding decisions in the first 6 weeks after birth', *Journal of Advanced Nursing*, vol. 66, no. 2, pp. 371–80.
4 Care Quality Commission (2013) *National Findings from the 2013 Survey of Women's Experiences of Maternity Care*, Newcastle upon Tyne: Care Quality Commission. Available at: www.cqc.org.uk/sites/default/files/media/documents/maternity_report_for_publication.pdf.
5 Sheehan, A., V. Schmied and L. Barclay (2010), pp. 371–80.
6 Telephone interview with Janet Fyle, 11 January 2014.
7 Sheehan, A., V. Schmied and L. Barclay (2010), pp. 371–80.
Furber, C. M. and A. M. Thomson (2008) 'Breastfeeding practice in the UK: midwives' perspectives', *Maternal and Child Nutrition*, vol. 4, no. 1, pp. 44–54.
Lagan, B. M., A. Symon, J. Dalzell and H. Whitford (2013) '"The midwives aren't allowed to tell you": perceived infant feeding policy restrictions in a formula feeding culture – the Feeding Your Baby study', *Midwifery*, vol. 30, no. 3, pp. e49–55, doi: 10.1016/j.miw.2013.10.017.
Lakshman, R., J. R. Landsbaugh, A. Schiff, S. Cohn, S. Griffing and K. K. Ong (2011) 'Developing a programme for healthy growth and nutrition during infancy: understanding user perspectives', *Child: Care, Health and Development*, vol. 38, no. 5, pp. 675–82, doi: 10.1111/j.1365-2214.2011.01283.x.
8 Lee, E. and F. Furedi (2005) *Mothers' Experience of, and Attitudes to, Using Infant Formula in the Early Months*, Canterbury: School of Social Policy, Sociology and Social Research, University of Kent. Available at: kar.kent.ac.uk/25249/1/Infant_Formula-Full[final].pdf.

9 Sheehan, A., V. Schmied and L. Barclay (2010), pp. 371–80.
10 Baby Friendly Hospital Initiative Australia (n.d.) 'Ten steps to successful breastfeeding'. Available at: www.babyfriendly.org.au/about-bfhi/ten-steps-to-successful-breastfeeding/ (accessed 20 December 2013).
11 UNICEF UK (n.d.) 'Baby Friendly Awards'. Available at: www.unicef.org.uk/ BabyFriendly/About-Baby-Friendly/Awards/ (accessed 20 December 2013).
12 Baby Friendly Hospital Initiative Australia (n.d.) 'Find a BFHI hospital'. Available at: www.babyfriendly.org.au/health-professionals/find-a-bfhi-hospital/.
13 Sheehan, A., V. Schmied and L. Barclay (2010), pp. 371–80.
14 Furber, C. M. and A. M. Thomson (2008), pp. 44–54.
    Barclay, L., J. Longman, V. Schmied, A. Sheehan, M. Rolfe, E. Burns and J. Fenwick (2012) 'The professionalisation of breast feeding: where are we a decade on?', Midwifery, vol. 28, no. 3, pp. 281–90.
    Chalmers, B. (2004) 'The Baby Friendly Hospital Initiative: where next?', BJOG, vol. 111, no. 3, pp. 198–9.
    Sheehan, A., V. Schmied and L. Barclay (2010), pp. 371–80.
15 Bartington, S., L. J. Griffiths, A. R. Tate, C. Dezateux and Millennium Cohort Study Child Health Group (2006) 'Are breastfeeding rates higher among mothers delivering in Baby Friendly accredited maternity units in the UK?', International Journal of Epidemiology, vol. 35, no. 5, pp. 1178–86. Available at: ije.oxfordjournals.org/content/35/5/1178.full.
16 UNICEF UK (n.d.) Moving from the Current to the New Baby Friendly Initiative Standards. London: UNICEF UK. Available at: www.unicef.org.uk/Documents/ Baby_Friendly/Guidance/transition_guidance.pdf.
17 McInnes, R. (2003) 'Commentary on original article "Mothers dealt with incompatible expectations during breast feeding and weaning" ', Evidence Based Nursing, vol. 6, no. 3, pp. 92. Available at: ebn.bmj.com/content/6/3/92. full.
18 Lagan, B. M. et al. (2013).
    Lakshman, R., D. Ogilvie and K. K. Ong (2009) 'Mothers' experiences of bottle-feeding: a systematic review of qualitative and quantitative studies', Archives of Disease in Childhood, vol. 94, no. 8, pp. 596–601.
    Labiner-Wolfe, J., S. B. Fein and K. R. Shealy (2008) 'Infant formula-handling education and safety', Pediatrics, vol. 122, supp. 2, pp. S85–90, doi: 10.1542/ peds.2008-1315k.
19 Lakshman, R. et al. (2009), pp. 596–601.
20 Furber, C. M. and A. M. Thomson (2008), pp. 44–54.
21 UNICEF UK (n.d.) 'Bottle feeding'. Available at: www.unicef.org.uk/BabyFriendly/ Health-Professionals/Care-Pathways/Bottle_feeding/First-days/Overview/.
22 Lee, E. and F. Furedi (2005), p. 4.
23 Lakshman, R. et al. (2011).
24 Battersby, S. (2010) 'An evaluation of midwives' knowledge of formula feeding and their role in supporting mothers who formula feed their infants', Journal of Family Health Care, vol. 20, no. 6, pp. 192–7.
25 Battersby, S. (2010), pp. 192–7.
26 Battersby, S. (2010), pp. 192–7.
27 In the UK, the Baby Milk Study, run by Cambridge University. Available at: www. mrc-epid.cam.ac.uk/research/studies/babymilk/. In Australia, a pilot study from the Queensland University of Technology.

28 Some quotes and ideas in this section first appeared in an article for *The Times* in July 2012. Morris, M. (2012) 'Breastfeeding is not always best', *The Times*, 31 July.

29 Telephone interview with Emma Shepherd, 16 June 2012.

30 Royal College of Psychiatrists (2012) 'Postnatal depression'. Available at: www. rcpsych.ac.uk/healthadvice/problemsdisorders/postnataldepression.aspx (accessed 9 January 2014).

31 Telephone interview with Dr Nicole Highet, 18 June 2012, citing as yet unpublished research.

32 Telephone interview with Dr Nicole Highet, 18 June 2012.

33 Haga, S. M., A. Lynne, K. Slinning and P. Kraft (2012) 'A qualitative study of depressive symptoms and well-being among first-time mothers', *Scandinavian Journal of Caring Sciences*, vol. 26, no. 3, pp. 458–66.

34 Telephone interview with Silje Marie Haga, 18 June 2012.

35 Telephone interview with Liz Wise, 19 June 2012.

36 Telephone interview with Rima Sidhpara, 18 June 2012.

37 Skype interview with Kate Kripke, 15 June 2012.

38 Feldman, R., A. Granat, C. Pariente, H. Kanety, J. Kurt and E. Gilboa-Schechtman (2009) 'Maternal depression and anxiety across the postpartum year and infant social engagement, fear regulation and stress reactivity', *Journal of the American Academy of Child and Adolescent Psychiatry*, vol. 48, no. 9, pp. 919–27.

39 Murray, L. (2006) 'The impact of postnatal depression on infant development', *Journal of Child Psychology and Psychiatry*, vol. 33, no. 3, pp. 543–61.

40 *Oxford English Dictionary*. Available at: www.oxforddictionaries.com/definition/ english/guilt?q=+guilt (accessed 28 November 2013).

41 William, K., N. Donaghue and T. Kurz (2012) ' "Giving guilt the flick"?: an investigation of mothers' talk about guilt in relation to infant feeding', *Psychology of Women Quarterly*, vol. 37, no. 1, pp. 97–112.

42 Liss, M., H. H. Schiffrin, V. H. Mackintosh, H. Miles-McLean and M. Erchull (2013) 'Development and validation of a quantitative measure of intensive parenting attitudes', *Journal of Child and Family Studies*, vol. 22, no. 5, pp. 621–36.

43 Skype interview with Professor David Lancy. For a very interesting, and reader-friendly, perspective on the history of childhood, I highly recommend Professor Lancy's blog 'Benign neglect' on *Psychology Today*. Particularly: www. psychologytoday.com/blog/benign-neglect/201202/detachment-parenting.

44 Bianchi, S. M., J. P. Robinson and M. A. Milkie (2006) *The Changing Rhythms of American Family Life*, New York: Russell Sage Foundation. This book relates to American family life but there is no reason to think it doesn't apply to other Western nations where the same sociological forces have been observed – more women working yet more intensive mothering.

45 Douglas, S. and M. Michaels (2004) *The Mommy Myth: The Idealization of Motherhood and How It Has Undermined All Women*, New York: The Free Press, p. 4.

46 This intensive mothering within a risk culture is something that Joan Wolf, the author of *Is Breast Best?*, calls 'total motherhood'. 'Total motherhood stipulates that mothers' primary occupation is to predict and prevent all less-than-optimal social, emotional, cognitive, and physical outcomes; that mothers are responsible for anticipating and eradicating every imaginable risk to their children, regardless of the degree or severity of the risk or what the trade-offs

might be; and that any potential diminution in harm to children trumps all other considerations in risk analysis as long as mothers can achieve the reduction.' Wolf, J. B. (2011) *Is Breast Best? Taking on the Breastfeeding Experts and the New High Stakes of Motherhood*, New York: New York University Press, p. 72.

47 Baby Center (2013) 'Which foods is my child most likely to be allergic to?' Available at: www.babycenter.com/404_which-foods-is-my-child-most-likely-to-be-allergic-to_10324755.bc (accessed 6 December 2013).

48 Parker-Pope, T. (2013) 'A surprising risk for toddlers on playground slides', *New York Times*, published online, 23 April. Available at: well.blogs.nytimes.com/2012/04/23/a-surprising-risk-for-toddlers-at-playground-slides/ (accessed 6 December 2013).

49 Dianne Wiessinger is also the author of the eighth edition of La Leche League's *Womanly Art of Breastfeeding*.

50 Wiessinger, D. (1996) 'Watch your language', *Journal of Human Lactation*, vol. 12, no. 1, pp. 1–4.

51 As quoted in Barston, S. (2012) *Bottled Up: How the Way We Feed Babies Has Come to Define Motherhood, and Why it Shouldn't*, Berkeley: University of California Press, p. 83.

52 *Oxford English Dictionary*. Available at: www.oxforddictionaries.com/definition/english/guilt?q=+guilt (accessed 28 November 2013).

53 This has been noted by many scholars, as detailed in Lee, E. (2011) *Feeding Babies and the Problems of Policy*, Canterbury: Centre for Parenting Culture Studies, University of Kent. Available at: blogs.kent.ac.uk/parentingculturestudies/files/2011/02/CPCS-Briefing-on-feeding-babies-FINAL-revised.pdf.

54 William, K., N. Donaghue and T. Kurz (2012), pp. 97–112.

55 Department for Transport (2012) *Reported Road Casualties in Great Britain: 2011 Annual Report*, London: Department for Transport. Available at: www.gov.uk/government/uploads/system/uploads/attachment_data/file/9273/rrcgb2011-00.pdf (accessed 9 December 2013).

56 Baby Center (2013) 'TVs toppling onto children at an alarming rate, study finds', 22 July. Available at: www.babycenter.com/204_tvs-toppling-onto-young-children-at-an-alarming-rate-study-f_10384900.bc?scid—omstodd_20130730:3&pe—IVCN0hmQnwyMDEzMDczMA.

57 Law, J. (2000) 'The politics of breastfeeding: assessing risk, dividing labor', *Signs*, vol. 25, no. 2, p. 415.

58 Moritz, M. L., M. D. Manole, D. L. Bogen and J. C. Ayus (2005) 'Breastfeeding-associated hypernatremia: are we missing the diagnosis?' *Pediatrics*, vol. 116, no. 3, pp. e343–7.

59 Rizzo, K. M., H. H. Schiffrin and M. Liss (2013) 'Insight into the parenting paradox: mental health outcomes of intensive mothering', *Journal of Childhood and Family Studies*, vol. 22, pp. 614–20.

60 This was strongly observed by Charlotte Faircloth of the Centre for Parenting Culture Studies at the University of Kent. 'One of the things that's quite interesting about parenting culture these days is that it doesn't encourage you to trust your own mother. So even if your mum does live around the corner, there's this sense that, well, she doesn't really know what she's talking about because, particularly in terms of the feeding, formula-feeding was more popular 30 years ago. So there's this sense that you should treat grandmothers with a bit of suspicion. They probably don't know the science, and that is quite an interesting

dynamic, because it's one of the first times that we question our parents.' Skype interview with Charlotte Faircloth, 21 November 2013.

61 Best for Babes (n.d.) 'What are the booby traps?' Available at: www. bestforbabes.org/what-are-the-booby-traps (accessed 11 December 2013).

62 Skype interview with Katie Hinde, 16 November 2013.

63 Baumslag, N. and D. L. Michels (1995) *Milk, Money and Madness: The Culture and Politics of Breastfeeding*, Westport: Bergin & Garvey, p. 93.

Part 2: The practice

1 Choosing a formula

1 Unless referenced otherwise, the vast majority of information in this chapter is sourced from: Crawley, H. and S. Westland (2013) *Infant Milks in the UK: A Practical Guide for Health Professionals*, London: First Steps Nutrition Trust. Available at: www.firststepsnutrition.org/pdfs/Infant_milks_June13.pdf.

2 WHO (2007) *Safe Preparation, Storage and Handling of Powdered Infant Formula: Guidelines*, Geneva: World Health Organization (WHO). Available at: www.who.int/foodsafety/publications/micro/pif_guidelines.pdf (accessed 1 January 2014).

3 NICE (2008) *Improving the Nutrition of Pregnant and Breastfeeding Mothers and Children in Low-income Households*, London: National Institute for Health and Clinical Excellence (NICE). Available at: www.nice.org.uk/nicemedia/pdf/ PH011guidance.pdf (accessed 29 December 2013).

4 Lozoff, B., M. Castillo, K. Clark and J. Smith (2011) 'Iron-fortified versus low-iron infant formula: developmental outcome at 10 years', *Archives of Pediatrics and Adolescent Medicine*, vol. 166, no. 3, pp. 208–15, doi: 10.1001/ archpediatrics.2011.197.

5 WHO (2007).

4 Preparing a feed

1 WHO (2007) *Safe Preparation, Storage and Handling of Powdered Infant Formula: Guidelines*, Geneva: World Health Organization (WHO). Available at: www.who.int/foodsafety/publications/micro/pif_guidelines.pdf (accessed 1 January 2014).

2 NHS Choices (2012) 'Can I use bottled water to make up baby formula (infant formula)?' Available at: www.nhs.uk/chq/Pages/1945.aspx?CategoryID=62&SubC ategoryID=64 (accessed 1 January 2014).

3 Victoria Department of Health (2011) *Young Infants, Infant Formula and Fluoride Exposure*, Melbourne: Department of Health. Available at: docs.health.vic.gov. au/docs/doc/92A62FAD09032AD2CA257868007ADB7B/$FILE/young_infant_ info_WEB_2011.pdf (accessed 2 January 2014).

5 Feeding

1 RCN (2013) *Formula Feeds: RCN Guidance for Nurses Caring for Infants and Mothers*, London: Royal College of Nursing (RCN). Available at: www.rcn.org. uk/__data/assets/pdf_file/0009/78741/003137.PDF (accessed 3 January 2014).

2 This table is based on the guidelines given by the First Steps Nutrition Trust. Crawley, H. and S. Westland (2013) *Infant Milks in the UK: A Practical Guide for*

Health Professionals, London: First Steps Nutrition Trust. Available at: www.
firststepsnutrition.org/pdfs/Infant_milks_June13.pdf.

6 Switching from breast to bottle

1 Thanks to Bottle Babies for their suggestions on this topic. See their guide on
introducing a bottle at www.bottlebabies.org/practical-support/how-tos-of-
bottle-feeding/how-to-get-baby-to-accept-the-bottle/.